REAL NURSES AND OTHERS

Racism in Nursing

Tania Das Gupta

Fernwood Publishing • Halifax & Winnipeg

To Esha Anum and Tara Saman

Editing: Brenda Conroy
Cover Design: John van der Woude
Printed and bound in Canada by Hignell Book Printing
Printed on paper containing 100% post-consumer fibre.

Published in Canada by Fernwood Publishing
32 Oceanvista Lane, Black Point, Nova Scotia, B0J 1B0
and #8 - 222 Osborne Street, Winnipeg, Manitoba, R3L 1Z3
www.fernwoodpublishing.ca

Fernwood Publishing Company Limited gratefully acknowledges the financial support of the Government of Canada through the Book Publishing Industry Development Program (BPIDP), the Canada Council for the Arts and the Nova Scotia Department of Tourism and Culture for our publishing program.

  Canadian Heritage / Patrimoine canadien   The Canada Council for the Arts / Le Conseil des Arts du Canada NOVA SCOTIA Tourism and Culture

Library and Archives Canada Cataloguing in Publication

Das Gupta, Tania, 1957-
Real nurses and others : racism in nursing / Tania Das Gupta.

Includes bibliographical references.
ISBN 978-1-55266-298-4

1. Discrimination in employment. 2. Discrimination in employment--Ontario. 3. Nurses--Employment. 4. Nurses--Employment--Ontario. 5. Race discrimination. 6. Race discrimination--Ontario. I. Title. II. Title: Racism in nursing.

RT83.3.D38 2009   331.13'3   C2008-907767-9

CONTENTS

ACKNOWLEDGEMENTS

I acknowledge financial and other assistance received from the Ontario Nurses' Association (ONA) in conducting this research. In particular, Karen Sandercock, Human Rights and Equity Specialist with ONA, provided me with ongoing feedback on drafts and was generous with her time and in facilitating access to relevant files, resource centres, members and relevant meetings. Without her support, this research would not have been possible.

I also acknowledge statistical services provided by the Institute of Social Research (ISR) at York University. The quantitative analysis provided by ISR greatly enhanced the value of my findings.

I extend my thanks to Dr. Rebecca Hagey for her assistance in distributing my survey to nurses and for her willingness to collaborate with me. Her sense of social justice and generosity made this project pleasurable and worthwhile.

I thank graduate students, including Kristin Blakely, Amrita Persaud, Monica Purdy and Ian McPhedran, who assisted me with extensive library searches or for conducting interviews with nurses.

Finally, I extend my thanks to all the nurses who shared their experiences, perspectives and insights. Their courage, tenacity and resourcefulness are truly inspiring.

PREFACE

My research into racism in nursing and, more specifically, into anti-Black racism in nursing is serendipitous. I had been researching racism in Canadian workplaces and I had always been interested in developing an intersectional analytical framework, focusing on race, gender and class relations. My first indepth look into this area was in relation to the garment industry in Toronto, which was the topic of my dissertation. At an activist level, I had worked with two high profile cases of racial harassment involving South Asian workers in Toronto, one involving food processing workers and the other involving steelworkers. Both were in non-unionized factories. Through these experiences, I could see how race, gender and class relations were used to disempower workers, by keeping them divided and also facilitating their exploitation.

In 1994, I was contacted by lawyers working with nurses at Toronto's Northwestern General Hospital (NWGH), from where seven nurses of colour had filed racial harassment complaints with the Ontario Human Rights Commission. All but one of these nurses were Black women. The seventh was a Filipino woman. The lawyers were looking for an academic who could provide them with some expertise in explaining how racism operated in NWGH. That was my entry into nursing. Subsequently, I worked with a number of different lawyers on a variety of cases mainly involving Black nurses who alleged racial harassment. It was through working on these actual cases that I developed many of my ideas that are contained in this book. Apparently, the analysis I had developed was found to be very useful by lawyers formulating their arguments. In my book *Racism and Paid Work* (1996), I included a chapter on nursing. The book has been widely used by university students and activists. Many workers of colour, including nurses, have told me that the book was enlightening and empowering for them because it articulated what they had been experiencing. It put their experiences into a language that they could understand and that made sense for them.

Encouraged by this positive response from readers, I wanted to do a larger study on this topic. The opportunity presented itself in 2000 when I was invited to speak on a panel organized by Ontario Nurses' Association (ONA), followed by a meeting of ONA's Racial Diversity Caucus. During the caucus meeting, I mentioned that I would be interested in conducting a study of systemic racism in nursing. Caucus members followed up on the idea and this book is the result. I hope that the research findings and the theoretical framework developed will be useful for nurses fighting racial harassment. Indeed, this book might be helpful for workers in any field confronted by racism.

1. WHY STUDY RACISM IN NURSING?

A couple of times, family would ask if I am the real nurse and I told them… RN means Real Nurse, something like that or I would say, they would think that I am… sort of like the health care aide or assistant. (Colleen)

About four years after she commenced work as an RN in Hospital "H," Joan was terminated. In her complaint filed at the Ontario Human Rights Commission, she said that events leading up to her dismissal led her to believe that she had been a victim of racial harassment and unequal treatment within her hospital on the basis of race and colour. Joan's complaint was filed against Hospital "H" as well as her nurse manager.

Joan worked in the chronic care unit, which, she noted, was largely staffed by Black nurses. Prior to working with the particular nurse manager who fired her, she had never had any problems with other nurse managers.

In the chronic care unit, Joan was frequently reminded about her lack of punctuality and cut in pay as a result, though her white counterparts were never subjected to similar treatment for being late. On one occasion she recalled her manager was unnecessarily critical of her regular nursing practices. The manager accompanied her during her rounds and reminded her of duties and responsibilities that were standard procedures. In addition, Joan recalled instances where she was asked to comment on what some of her Black colleagues had said or done. Her feeling was that information was being gathered in this manner in order to use it to their detriment. She noted that she had never been asked to comment on any white colleagues.

After one particularly confrontational interaction between Joan and her manager over the issue of being late, a claim disputed by Joan, she went home for being too upset to continue working. She was then suspended from work without pay for two days. On her first day back, Joan was met by her manager and accused of a variety of things, including tardiness, leaving early, misuse of a hospital phone, refusing to put patients in and out of bed, yelling and a number of other actions. Joan received a termination letter. She pointed out that she had been fired without due process, such as formal warnings. She filed a grievance through the Ontario Nurses' Association (ONA). (Das Gupta 1996b: 101)

For over a decade, a number of labour and human rights lawyers have found it necessary to consult with me on cases similar to the one cited above in order to prepare arguments of racial harassment against hospital management. Most of the affected people have been Black women working as registered nurses in Ontario. The fact that these lawyers have to resort to calling me (an academic) to establish the merits of their cases demonstrates that complainants such as Joan are not readily believed by arbitrators, tribunals and judges. The situation of these complainants is much like that of an assaulted or raped woman who is not believed. The perpetrator is assumed innocent unless proven guilty. The onus is on the victim to prove that she has indeed been violated. Feminists have argued that this process further victimizes the woman as she has to not only establish the fact of being violated but also to prove that she is honest and that she did not invite the attack (Welsh et al. 2001). Underlying the imperative to prove her credibility are certain assumptions about women being responsible for the attack by somehow tempting or provoking the men who rape them. Certain historically derived discourses around gender relations and notions of femininity and masculinity are invoked each time a woman comes forward with a charge of assault or rape against a man. These invocations influence the responses and actions taken by policymakers, police officers, counsellors, healthcare workers and sometimes even her relatives and loved ones.

Some progress has been made in educating the public about the experience of sexual harassment and rights of women, thanks to the work of feminists. As a result, the criminal justice system, including the police, has been directed to be much more proactive in charging rapists and those who commit violence against women. In theory, at least, women who are attacked and give evidence of having experienced it are to be believed and supported. In practice, of course, victims of violence are still not always protected by society, particularly when they are Aboriginal women, immigrant women or women of colour. In the case of racial harassment, however, it appears that even the theoretical departure from past practice has not happened. Workers who bring forward cases of racial harassment, particularly if they are Black women and men, are almost always assumed to be exaggerating their complaints, to "have a chip on their shoulder" or "to be playing the race card" in order to cover up their deficiencies and personal shortcomings. Moreover, they are seen to be "subjective" and therefore not believable. An outside academic is brought in, on the assumption that he or she is completely "objective." Just as the discounting of an injured party as subjective and thus unreliable is problematic, so is the reliance on the academic as objective and therefore reliable. Knowledge is never completely objective as who we are and our social location condition our vantage point and the aspects of reality that we can see and theorize on. Be that as it may, the practice of discounting the words of those subjected to racial harassment continues. The onus is on the victim to prove it. This book is an attempt to reverse this dynamic so that society becomes more educated about how workplace racial harassment functions, particularly in the Canadian context.

The time is right to prioritize the addressing of racism and racial harassment. It is an urgent matter across the country, but particularly so in cities such as Toronto. A focus on Toronto is therefore useful in pointing out these realities, which may be relevant for other urban centres as well. The Ethnic Diversity Survey (Statistics Canada 2003) conducted by Statistics Canada in conjunction with the Department of Canadian Heritage in 2002 revealed that 13 percent of Canadian population aged fifteen or older, accounting for 2.9 million people, were people of colour.[1] The most frequent origins were Chinese and South Asian (Statistics Canada 2003). Most live in Toronto, Vancouver or Montreal. In fact, some municipalities have half or a majority of residents consisting of people of colour, for instance, 59 percent of Richmond, B.C., 55 percent of Markham, Ontario, and 50 percent each of Vancouver and Burnaby, B.C. The non-white population is growing six times faster than the rest of the population.

Within this demographic context, people of colour were more likely than others to say that they felt uncomfortable or out of place in Canada because of their ethnicity, culture, race, skin colour, accent, language or religion (Statistics Canada 2003: 19). Of all the people who expressed this sentiment, 56 percent said that they had experienced this at work or when applying for work. These realities indicate that although most Canadians are living comfortably with their diverse ethnic/racial origins, a significant proportion is not. If Aboriginal people and people of mixed racial origins were included in the counting, the problem would be even larger. This presents a challenge for us as citizens, educators and policymakers, indeed as employers, unions and community groups.

Universal healthcare is as Canadian as ice hockey or maple syrup. Canadians feel a sense of pride about their achievements in this area not only because it is held up as an example of the social welfare state in Canada, but because it is something that differentiates us from our neighbour to the south, the United States of America. In recent years, deteriorating conditions in healthcare have led to a great deal of anxiety about the erosion of this element of our identity. Popular discourse has pointed out the long waiting lines in emergency units of hospitals, the plundering of the system by fraudulent members of the public, the closure of hospitals and the spectre of privatized healthcare ushering in a dual-tiered system, one for the rich and another for the poor. What is not readily apparent in this discourse is the racial aspect — that among those potentially most disenfranchised from the deteriorating healthcare system in Canada are people of colour, Aboriginal people, immigrants and refugees, women, people with disabilities and people who are poor and/or homeless. This disenfranchisement not only takes the forms of exclusion, unemployment and underemployment, but also harassment on the job.

Focusing on racism in hospitals and related healthcare settings gives us a glimpse of the complexity of this issue as it is manifested in social situations marked by human vulnerability.[2] How does one negotiate power relationships and stand up for one's rights in a setting where both perpetrator and victim may be dealing with a seriously ill or dying person? In some cases, the perpetrator may be ill or dying. Moreover, interactions in these settings may take place in intimate relations and resemble those that take place within the family. Harassment in this context resembles abuse in familial situations. Does the vulnerability of the perpetrator, either as a patient or as a caregiver, shield her from retaliation or resistance by the victim of racism? How does the vulnerability of the receiver/victim as a worker within the nursing hierarchy affect her ability to resist or to retaliate? What ethical dilemmas does it raise for her? How does harassment make her even more vulnerable? Moreover, what if prolonged racial harassment is causing the receiver to become sick or disabled?

In the cases brought to my attention, it is difficult to establish the fact of racial harassment as the women complainants bear no physical scars or any other evidence of being physically damaged by the harassment. It is reminiscent of emotional abuse suffered by women in intimate relationships. It is noteworthy though that advocates have noted that those subjected to prolonged racial harassment invariably suffer from psycho-somatic illnesses, such as ulcers, depression and insomnia. Working in a "poisoned environment" (Ontario Women's Directorate 1994: 6) is believed to be the cause of these ailments (see also Feagin 2003; Hagey et al. 2001; Edmonds 2001; McKenzie 2003; Kirchheimer 2003). Studies have shown that racism is a hazard to the health of people of colour, and it has been argued that racism in the workplace is a health and safety issue. In recognition of this principle, the Canadian Union of Public Employees (CUPE) Local One, at Ontario Hydro (now known as Toronto Hydro), negotiated an anti-harassment policy, which allows workers alleging harassment under the Ontario Human Rights Code to leave their workplace without loss of pay, just as workers can refuse to work in an unsafe environment under Ontario's health and safety legislation (CUPE Manual).

This study also illustrates the complexity of racism in the workplace as it cross-cuts gender and class discrimination. Thus, power emanates in these settings not only on the basis of racialization, but also on the basis of one's location within the workplace hierarchy as well as one's gender. Being a woman imposes certain social expectations on a nurse and being a woman of colour further complicates the situation. Nursing by its very nature is associated with women's labour within the family, as alluded to before. Her work includes feeding (food and medicines), attending, healing, nurturing and bodily cleaning and is subordinate to the work of physicians. The latter are associated with long and expensive levels of education to train them to perform complicated surgeries, prescribe medication and provide diagnosis and treatment plans. This work is considered "mental" and male, even though there are more females in the medical profession than in years past. Heterosexist family ideologies operate in these settings, where doctors are "father" figures, while nurses are "mother" figures, and patients are akin to children and other dependents within families. How does racialization mark these familial dynamics? Are women of colour viewed as "maids" and "servants" — as "outsiders within"? The opening excerpt in this chapter from Colleen, a Black nurse, points in this direction. She talks about how her authenticity as a registered nurse (RN) was regularly questioned by patients, who often assumed that she was in a lower category of nursing, namely a healthcare aide or a nursing assistant, because her blackness identified her in a lower social rung, a position where she would be assisting or serving "real" (white) nurses.

As mentioned before, I work with lawyers who contact me for help with the preparation of their cases on racial harassment in the workplaces, mostly involving Black nurses. In my capacity as an academic advisor and "expert," I worked with the Ontario Nurses' Association[3] (ONA), and in November 2000 I was invited to speak on a panel concerning human rights issues at its Equity Caucuses Meeting. At the conclusion of this meeting, ONA's Racially Diverse Caucus brought forward the recommendation that ONA conduct research into racism in nursing. Subsequently, an agreement was reached with ONA that I would undertake a one-year exploratory study of racism in nursing in Ontario. The study was planned at the end of 2001 and conducted in 2002.

The study was exploratory in that the initial objective was to lay bare the common experiences, patterns, features and surface manifestations of systemic racism in nursing in Ontario. However, anyone who has done research on "race" and racism knows that people do not readily talk about racism, neither do they identify their experiences as being those of racism. It quickly became apparent that in order to make sense of personal experiences and testimonies, one has to understand the ways in which systemic racism works, that is, understand the features that are frequently not revealed through personal observations, and to identify the linkages between disparate experiences, events, policies, procedures and practices. This requires theorizing, developing a conceptual understanding of what racism is and how it works. Hence, the second objective of this study was to develop a theoretical framework for understanding systemic racism. It is hoped that this framework is relevant for analyzing racism in any workplace or occupation and will become an educational and organizing tool for workers in any site.

This book, which is based on the report of my study but which goes beyond it, has seven chapters. The two chapters following this introductory chapter are of a theoretical nature. In Chapter 2, I elaborate on my definitions of racism and present a framework for understanding how different forms of racism work and are connected to each other. This discussion, titled "Theorizing Racism, Gender and Class: Concepts, Theories and Histories," also demonstrates how racism works in concert with other forms of oppression, such as sexism and classism. It lays the foundations for a theoretical framework that is developed later on to understand racism specifically in healthcare and nursing.

Chapter 3, titled "Political Economy of Healthcare: Class, Race and Gender Perspectives," contextuates racism in nursing within an understanding of the larger economic and political relationships framing healthcare in Canada. For instance, a predominant characteristic of healthcare in the 1980s and 1990s was that of restructuring. Restructuring has to be seen within a larger neo-liberal policy direction in which the Canadian state cut back its resource contributions, rationalized by a rhetoric of "fiscal crisis," "efficiency" and "eliminating wastage." This had a profound impact on those who were employed in healthcare, particularly on women, immigrants and people of colour, the most vulnerable sections of the working population. The third chapter also includes the methodologies used to conduct this study.

Chapters 4, 5 and 6 present my research findings. Since I used a variety of techniques, I was able to acquire diverse information on how racism expresses itself in the paid workplace. Thus, each of these chapters throws light on how systemic racism operates from an experiential, institutional and discursive perspective. In Chapter 4, I present a case study of one nurse of colour whose work experiences embody the entire cycle of racism, from everyday racism to behavioural forms at the hands of her managers and co-workers to more systemic forms and finally at a cultural level with common-sensical expressions of how she was perceived as a Black woman.

In Chapter 5, I present the results of a survey I conducted with 593 ONA members, both white and non-white, with regard to their experience of workplace racism. The quantified results are powerful indications of the extent of the problem and its common features. These results are presented in conjunction with excerpts from indepth interviews conducted with nurses, as well as information gleaned from arbitration reports, which I was able to review from ONA files.

Chapter 6 provides a discourse analysis of racism as it was expressed by nurses on the survey forms in the form of "comments." The discourses identified are discussed in the context of sociological writings on new racism today, which operates without using the word "race."

The concluding chapter identifies major findings, themes, policy implications, research limitations and areas for future research. It also provides an update of what happened with the report generated out of the study.

NOTES

1. This does not include the Aboriginal population. Neither does it include mixed ethnic/racial heritages. If these groups were included also, the number would be even higher
2. This point emerged in conversation with Dr. Carl James, a colleague and noted anti-racism scholar at York University, Toronto, Canada.
3. Founded in 1973, the Ontario Nurses' Association (ONA) is the trade union that represents 48,000 registered nurses and allied health professionals working in hospitals, long-term care facilities, public health, community agencies and industry throughout Ontario.

2. THEORIZING RACISM, GENDER AND CLASS
Concepts, Theories and Histories

Since this book focuses on racism, it is appropriate to delve in as much detail as possible into the nature of this topic, particularly as it manifests itself in the labour market and in paid work sites. As will become evident, the problematic nature of issues and concepts related to racism and salient debates involving these concepts make it quite challenging to conduct research in this area, particularly in its material manifestations. This chapter first discusses some of the debates in the theorizing of "race," racism and related issues. Second, it throws light on racism in Canada, with emphasis on the economic sphere and with particular reference to African/Black Canadians. Third, it looks at the intersectional nature of social relations, including those involving racialization, and explores how racialization processes intersect with class and gender relations.

"RACE," RACISM AND RACIALIZATION

There is considerable debate among social scientists on what "race" is all about and whether the term should be used at all. For instance, Miles and Torres (1996) argue that "race" is not a valid sociological concept because the idea that human beings can be categorized into discrete "races," "each exhibiting a set of physical and cultural characteristics," has been proven false by genetic and biological sciences (Montagu 1951). Further, they argue, continuing to use it as a concept despite its rejection validates and perpetuates "race" thinking. One indication of that is that complex social phenomena continue to be attributed to one's position within racial categories. Miles and Torres, therefore, insist on referring to the "idea of race" only in quotation marks to denote its problematic nature and never employing it as a theoretical concept. On the other hand, Omi and Winant (1994: 1) argue that "race has been a profound determinant of one's political rights, one's location in the labour market, and indeed one's sense of 'identity.'" Arguing for the "irreducible political aspect of racial dynamics," they assert the "social nature of race, the absence of any essential racial characteristics" and the "historical flexibility of racial meanings and categories." However, Miles and Torres argue that the sheer use of the word in an unproblematic way has the effect of "re-inventing and re-ritualizing" it, and they illustrate how the word and its associated meanings offer an explanation of social reality, albeit in incomplete and unsatisfactory forms.

In Canada, Castagna and Dei (2000) argue that "race" exists materially, politically, socially and ideologically in the lives of people and therefore one cannot dismiss it as a social construct only. Moreover, apart from the issue of how race was constructed originally, it is constantly being reformulated in specific contexts to accommodate particular historical events, cultures and resistances. Moreover, the authors (2000: 20) argue that the reality of skin colour racism cannot be denied and in fact far outweighs the virulence of other forms of racism. They state: "While the reproduction of racism can be rooted in contemporary social, political and economic forces, the production of racism may well lie beyond these forces, extending to an ideology that supports white supremacy for its own sake, without being driven by economic interests necessarily" (19). They continue to consider "the race concept" as having usefulness. As Miles (1989) suggests, many scholars have conflated "race," racism and racist structures and this problem has reduced the rigour with which racism has been analyzed and resisted.

While skin colour racism is undeniably present in Canada and other Western European societies, particularly in paid workplaces, there is a danger that in holding it up as "the primary" or the "harshest" form of racism, one can obfuscate other forms of racism, those based on or intersecting with issues of religion, language, culture or nationalism, often referred to as "new racism" (Gilroy 2000: 34). This is particularly illustrated by post-9/11 racism against Arabs (in particular Muslims) in Western societies, or those perceived to be Arabs and Muslims (according to predominant stereotypes), such as South Asians (Sikh, Hindu or Muslim), some of whom could be described as "white" or "brown" skinned. In such cases, the "other" is marked not always by brown or black skin, but rather with "darker" facial hair, "Asian" sounding names, turbans, hijabs, shalwar kameezes or other signifiers of being of an otherized religious group, namely Muslims. Similar illustrations of racism against people who appear "white" include anti-Semitism against Jews in Western societies, racism against Roma people in Europe, against displaced persons (DPs) from the Ukraine in Canada in the early 1920s and against French-Canadians. Moreover, the formulation of a primacy of skin colour-based racism, which inevitably posits a dichotomy of experience between whites and non-whites, does not throw light on intra-ethnic racism, i.e., racism within and among people of colour themselves, such as that based on ethnic and religious differences or degrees of "darkness." Omi and Winant (1994: 73) and Miles and Torres (1996: 35) recognize the need to acknowledge that racism is not only a white monopoly, that non-whites can be racist too.

My position in this debate is one marked by contradiction, but I hope not confusion. I hold that people's constructed differences based on skin colour, culture, religion, language and other features are utilized to slot them into different racial categories, which result in inequalities and oppressions in all facets of their lives. There may be a debate over the idea of "race" and whether to use the term or not, but there is consensus on the reality of racism in people's lives based on the "idea of race" and the processes of racialization, the latter being a concept elaborated by Miles (1989: 73–77). My use of the term "race" is limited, following on Miles and Torres' rationale; however, I do use it in my formulation of questions to nurses in this study to document how and why they are subjected to differential and inferior treatment in their workplaces as a result of the idea of "race" and their subsequent racialization. In order to "get at" the effects of racism at their work sites, I do have to rely on a language of "race." Hence, there is an inherent contradiction in my work in that, while theoretically I subscribe wholeheartedly to Miles and Torres' argument, I do rely on "race" talk to get at the ways in which racism results in material inequalities among workers on the basis of their racialization. Moreover, this dilemma is shared by many "anti-racists," whose efforts are based on "race" discourses and amount to racial projects (Omi and Winant 1994: 72). A good example is that of affirmative action, which relies on counting bodies based on their "race" status and then insists that representation of bodies in any organization should reflect the range of racialized bodies in the available population outside the organization. Omi and Winant differentiate between the essentialism inherent in racist ideologies and "strategic" essentialism practised by members of inferiorized groups. Benjamin (2003) expounds the concept of strategic essentialism further by saying that this type of essentialism is defined by the marginalized group itself rather than its oppressors. Further, "the group rather paradoxically acknowledges that such attributes are not natural (or intrinsically essential), but are merely invoked when it is politically useful to do so" (83). In contrast, Gilroy (2000) makes an appeal to critical scholars in racism to reflect on this dilemma and make a departure from a "race discourse." My particular utilization of the term "race" in my research puts me closer to Omi and Winant (1994) and Benjamin (2003).

RACISM AS AN IDEOLOGY

Miles (1989) refers to the ideology of racism or "racialism" when he discusses late eighteenth- and nineteenth-century "scientific" writings on "race." Before that period, Miles says that discussions of the "other" were not based on "race" and therefore did not constitute racism, but rather ethnocentrism. Moreover, Miles differentiates between the ideology of racism and "exclusionary practice," between "cognition and action." According to him, ideology must be distinguished by "its content rather than by its function." It has two components: first, some biological or cultural characteristic that identifies a group as being of a distinct category or "race," which is inherent and unchangeable, and second, that the distinguishing biological or cultural characteristics are represented as contributing to the group's inferiority. Miles further argues that the ideology of racism does not only arise out of scientific or logical arguments around "race" thinking but also from a "less coherent assembly of stereotypes, images, attributions, and explanations." Together, the content of racism as it presents itself at any time provides an explanation of the lived realities of people.

My understanding of racism is similar to Miles', i.e., as an ideology or a discourse that differentiates between people on the basis of outward physical characteristics, such as skin colour, hair texture and facial features, and then evaluates their intellectual and cultural characteristics as being inferior or superior on the basis of these superficial characteristics. Non-traditional (non-European) headdresses, hairstyles, beards or moustaches, or modes of dressing and jewellery, can also become physical markers of difference from the white norm. Indeed, difference is often constructed based on sheer imagination or the desire to draw a protective barrier against people who appear to be physically different from oneself. For instance, according to Miles (1989), during the Middle Ages, the Greco-Roman world imagined whole populations as *monstra*, i.e., as monsters, to represent them as outsiders. White male European eugenicists of the late eighteenth century defined racial superiority and its converse, inferiority, based on such things as the shape or size of different body parts, including the head, the nose, the ears, the buttocks and sexual organs, criteria that have now been concluded to be invalid, although some still continue to uphold them as "science." Moreover, Gilroy (2000) has argued that there is a "re-birth" of a new kind of biological racism, one based on "cellular and molecular, not dermal" sciences (47). Racism involves a process of racialization (Miles 1989: 75), where meaning is attributed to physical (or "somatic" according to Miles), cultural, religious and other bodily markers so that individuals are viewed and defined as being members of discrete "races." Miles says, "the concept therefore refers to a process of categorization, a representational process of defining an Other..." (75). Moreover, it is a gendered process as racial categories are considered as "discrete breeding population[s]." The process of racialization is historically specific, so that the meaning given to bodily features vary over time and space, and what is most overt depends on a range of political, economic, social and other factors. Thus, one can talk about many different racisms, all of which co-exist and intersect with each other. Authors have named anti-Black racism, Islamophobia, anti-Semitism, Orientalism, to name a few forms. Thus, a person who is a Black Jew is likely to be affected by the first and third forms mentioned; a Hindu South Asian might be marginalized within an Orientalist discourse, and so on.

ATTITUDINAL, EVERYDAY AND BEHAVIOURAL RACISM

Omi and Winant (1994: 74) state that authors have debated as to whether racism is "primarily an ideological or structural phenomenon." As mentioned before, Miles maintains that exclusionary practices could be happening for a number of different reasons and their connection with racist ideology must be demonstrated rather than assumed. Similarly, exclusionary practices or processes could be intentional or unintentional, unlike the intentionally negative evaluation of a racialized collectivity.

Unlike Miles, however, I do not restrict my understanding of racism only to the realm of representation or cognition. In my view, racism includes a number of related elements including attitudes (prejudices and stereotypes), behaviours or practices (individual and institutional) and ideologies (theories and common sense). The latter has been discussed by Lawrence (2004) and Miles (1989). In addition, "everyday" racism, as developed by Essed (1991), is also part of my framework. While Miles has argued that scholars discussing racism have contributed to "conceptual inflation" by referring to all of these varying components, I maintain that one does not have to conceptually conflate them, but rather recognize their inter-relationship and mutual reinforcement and that they constitute a formation, sometimes with internal contradictions.

I argue that these different aspects of racism, including racialization, its ideological content, its everyday, common-sensical forms, as well as its associated processes and practices are all connected and are important towards developing a comprehensive and complex understanding of racism. So for example, everyday racism is socially constructed by individual behaviours, social interactions and common-sensical beliefs held by individuals, which originate in racist ideologies received from the past. Moreover, this process is enabled within institutions that operate with policies and practices that are racist in effect, i.e., they disadvantage those who are seen as "others" or "outsiders."

In this framework, the transition from the everyday form to the trans-historical discursive form is fluid and simultaneous. As Essed (1991) theorizes, the micro and the macro levels, the cognitive and structural forms of racism, occur simultaneously. Omi and Winant's concepts of "racial formation" and "racial project" are useful in making sense of the complexity of racism:

> An alternative approach is to think of racial formation processes as occurring through a linkage between structure and representation. Racial projects do the ideological "work" of making these links. *A racial project is simultaneously an interpretation, representation, or explanation of racial dynamics, and an effort to re-organize and redistribute resources along particular racial lines.* Racial projects connect what race *means* in a particular discursive practice and the ways in which both social structures and everyday experiences are racially *organized* based upon that meaning. (1994: 56, emphasis in original)

In summary, they state that debates about whether racism is primarily ideological or structural are not helpful by arguing that "ideological beliefs have structural consequences and that social structures give rise to beliefs."

EVERYDAY RACISM AS RACIST BEHAVIOUR

The dynamics of the "everyday" is crucial in understanding how racism is experienced. Everyday "ambiguous" or "conflictual" thinking is related to everyday behaviours, which is where racism is most frequently encountered by people of colour. Moreover, it is difficult to identify the structures and ideologies of everyday racism if one looks only at individual incidents. Interactions may include a few words exchanged, words not exchanged, gestures, glances, tone of voice, rumours, coincidences, inclusions and exclusions, which individually seem odd but not overtly problematic. However, considered collectively, they reveal a pattern of marginalization and differential treatment of non-whites. Taken individually, they seem minute and thus cannot readily be classified as racism. However, they are the form of racism that people of colour face every day. Essed (1991: 47) defines everyday racism as

> a process in which (a) socialized racist notions are integrated into meanings that make practices immediately definable and manageable, (b) practices with racist implications become in themselves familiar and repetitive, and (c) underlying racial and ethnic relations are actualized and reinforced through these routine or familiar practices in everyday situations.

Essed discusses everyday racism in the forms of underestimation, enforcement of cultural assimilation and pathologization of Blacks. If we analyze these practices, we find that they are expressions of "race" thinking, which reproduce existing race and ethnic relations in society.

Everyday racism is not a continuous experience. In the context of racism experienced by Blacks in the Netherlands, Essed argues that Black workers have non-racist experiences also; however, certain situations take on a racial tone. We could say that they become racialized. Everyday racism usually takes a behavioural form, something that is said, not said, done or not done by a member of the racially dominant group.

Omi and Winant discuss everyday experience as an aspect of racial formation. They envoke the concept of "common sense" to connect racist beliefs with everyday perception, comments and interactions. For example, they refer to the ways in which we "notice" the "race" of people we encounter and if someone is not neatly defined into a racialized category, a sense of disorientation often results. Similarly, experiences and interactions are racialized just as we learn to racialize people. Race becomes "common sense." They argue that we learn about "race" ideology unconsciously and it becomes a way in which we go about our daily business. In conducting research on racism, therefore, it often becomes necessary to use the language of "race" to ask workers about their experiences of racism, and herein lies the dilemma of reinscribing "race" as an ideology.

NEW RACIAL FORMATIONS

A number of social scientists have discussed the complexities of "de-racialization" of racist behaviour and discourse in contemporary times (Billig et al. 1988; Henry et al. 2000; Jakubowski 1997). Billig et al. (1988) talk about ambivalence and ambiguity in racial discourse where attitudes about people of colour are expressed indirectly, politely and reasonably. In this new discourse of race, people of colour are negatively reflected upon because they, their behaviours and activities, cultures and equity policies are evaluated as challenging liberal values of equality, freedom and fairness. This is reminiscent of workplace discourses where so-called "incompetence" or "lack of professionalism" are often invoked to evaluate, discipline or dismiss workers of colour. White people acting in these ways maintain that they are not prejudiced or racist. Often, this takes the form of what Van Dijk (1993) calls "an 'on the one hand' and 'on the other hand' strategy." For example, a white person says, "one the one hand, I'm not racist, but on the other hand workers of colour are lowering the standards." Billig et al. (1988) note that this ambivalence and ambiguity about racism reflects an ideological dilemma, one between intellectual ideology and lived ideology. I suggest that the two latter concepts seem parallel to the concepts of ideology versus common sense in Gramsci's writings. "Lived ideology" according to Billig et al. (1988), "refers to ideology as a society's way of life." This sort of ideology includes what passes for common sense within a society. "Intellectual ideology" is a system of political, religious or philosophical thinking and, as such, is very much the product of intellectuals or professional thinkers (27). Billig et al. further clarify that lived ideology is synonymous with the notion of "culture" or "everyday thinking." The problem with Billig et al.'s argument is that it posits everyday thinking or culture as racist while assuming that intellectual forms of ideology are racially neutral. On the contrary, Jakubowski (1997: 44) maintains, using J. Reeves' writings, that laws and policies that appear to be formal, intellectual and coherent are not neutral at all. She illustrates how so-called de-racialized language in legal and political discourses hides racism through the use of rhetorical devices, such as equivocation. The latter technique of using "vague" or "misleading" terms to make the meaning am-biguous or confusing allows racist ideas to be communicated privately within a public discourse that appears non-racist. The example used to illustrate this technique is the phrase "controlling immigration," which on its surface appears de-racialized, but can have a private connotation of "controlling the entry of non-whites into the country."

Racially ambivalent feelings have been analyzed by Katz et al. (1986) and Dovidio and Gaertner (1986), who note that white Americans face a conflict of core values, one representing egalitarianism and the other representing individualism and meritocracy. Thus, while many whites might support de-segregation and equal opportunity programs to address racism, they might oppose state imposed mandatory busing to alter segregated schools and quota systems that accompany an affirmative action program. Dovidio and Gaertner (1986) add that this ambivalence is not only due to a conflict in core values, but also to negative feelings and beliefs about Black Americans that are part and parcel of American culture. These conflicts result in certain types of behaviour in whites, particularly avoidance of Blacks. Attitudinal surveys reveal ambiguous responses from white Americans vis-à-vis racism. Whether one calls this kind of racism "new," "aversive," "symbolic" or "democratic" (Henry et al. 2000), the salient point is that today's racism often has a differ-ent discourse from old-fashioned racism, which makes it difficult to identify and prevent in society, including the workplace.

SYSTEMIC RACISM, INSTITUTIONAL RACISM AND RACIST DISCOURSE

I describe systemic racism as arising

> from conscious or unconscious policies, procedures and practices which adversely affect people of colour, such as their exclusion, marginalization and infantilization. Systemic racism is supported by institutional power, i.e. by the allocation of resources, codification of "standard" policies and procedures, and by workplace environ-ment. Therefore, systemic racism is perpetuated over time. (Das Gupta 1996a: 12).

Although Miles (1989) does not discuss "systemic" racism *per se*, he does address another related aspect of racism, namely "institutional" racism. Interestingly enough, in his discussion of the latter, he brings together the dimensions of racism as practice and as discourse, an intersection that he argued earlier contributed to conceptual conflation. However, he insists that the intersection between discourse and practice in this case must be demon-strated rather than assumed. According to him, institutional racism arises in two situations: first where a set of practices that originally arose out of racially exclusionary intentions currently continue without the discursive rationale underpinning it; second, where the original discourse has dissipated and a new discourse, often de-racialized to suit the current rules of acceptability, continues and supports racially exclusionary practices. Miles insists that what defines institutional racism is not the "effect" of exclusionary practice but rather a link between the practices and explicitly racist discourse. He offers the example of the blatant exclusion of Asian and Black immigrants from Britain openly demanded by white Britishers in the 1950s being implemented through the 1968 *Commonwealth Immigrants Act* and the 1971 *Immigration Act* on the pretext that "immigration control" was "good for race relations" (85–86). My conceptualization of systemic racism is very similar to Miles' conceptualization of institutional racism; however, unlike the latter, I bring together both the effects of exclusionary practices and a racist discourse underpinning it.

Many of the leading anti-racism theorists argue that racism exists in "articulation" (Miles 1989; Calliste and Dei 2000) with other social relations, such as those of gender, class and nation. Specifically, the articulation of racialization with gender and class has been developed by feminists of colour and is sometimes referred to as the "race, gender and class" approach.

RACE, GENDER AND CLASS APPROACH

The race, gender and class approach is also referred to as "anti-racist feminism" (Dua and Robertson 1999), "intersectional theorizing" (Stasiulis 1999), the "matrix of domination" (Hill and Collins 1990: 222) and "integrative anti-racism" (Dei 1998: 306). Dua (1999) argues that there are a number of different approaches in how anti-racist feminism has advanced in Canada. This was a development of feminism, particularly from the perspective of feminists of colour. One variant (Ng 2002; Bannerji 1995) of this approach has been to build on Dorothy Smith's (1992) methodology of beginning from the lived realities of women, in this case women of colour, to lay bare their embodiment of the social relations that affect them. This is referred to as "standpoint methodology." Anti-racist feminism has also been developed using a political economy approach that includes anti-racist analysis (Stasiulis 1999; Das Gupta 1996b). This second group of theorists argues that discourses of race operate within a capitalist framework. Their starting point is different in that standpoint feminism begins with the everyday and everynight experiences of immigrant women and women of colour, which are gendered, classed and raced, and then connects how that is socially organized within capitalist institutions and racist discourse. The latter group begins from the larger context of the capitalist political economy, which is raced, classed and gendered, and analyzes how immigrant women and women of colour are located within that structure. What is common to both the standpoint anti-racist feminists and the political economy anti-racist feminists is the understanding that our experiences are complex as they are simultaneously shaped by multiple and intersecting power relations. The anti-racist feminist approach was mainly developed by feminists of colour in Canada, such as Bannerji (1995), Ng (2006), Dua (1999), Das Gupta (1996b) and elsewhere, such as Hill Collins

(1990), and hooks (1992), to name just a few writers who critique traditional feminist paradigms and movements as focusing solely on gender oppression, which do not capture the experiences of women of colour. They argue that most women of colour not only face gender oppression, but also that of racism, class exploitation and heterosexism. Thus feminist theory needs to be more inclusive of other forms of oppression that affect women of colour, working class women, women with disabilities and lesbians. Moreover, they posit that no form of oppression is primary as they operate simultaneously, affecting individuals in contradictory or complementary ways. They are described as "intersecting" and "interlocking."

The ways in which power relations affect us depends on where each of us is located within society, that is, within race relations, class relations, gender relations and other sets of social relations. Thus, identities and positions of race, gender, class, sexuality, etc. are socially constructed relationally, so that "men" are considered "masculine" in relation to "women" or what is "feminine" within a particular society. A person who is considered "white" in any society is defined in relation to who is considered "not white" or a "person of colour." Thus, non-whites, females, workers, homosexuals, people with disabilities are looked upon as the "other" or the deviant in relation to the "self," which is defined as white, male, middle/upper class, heterosexual, able-bodied and "normal." Moreover, these discourses intersect and influence each other. For example, McClintock (1995: 52–56) discusses how working-class white women and Irish men and women were represented as inferior races in the context of British imperialism. This characterization depicted their deviance from the white upper-class norm. Conversely, men and women of colour were represented as feminized and masculinized respectively in order to convey their racial degeneration and deviance. The ability to define and represent individuals in this manner and to prefer one over the other is a result of power relations that exist between those who define and those who are defined (hooks 1992), between those who are materially in control and those who are not, between those who have everyday privileges and those who do not. What these representations show us also is that hegemonic definitions of masculinity, femininity, whiteness, Blackness or other racialized, sexualized and gendered categories are subject to social construction and are fairly arbitrary. Moreover, a person may be in dominance in one set of social relations, such as gender, but be subordinate in another set of social relations, such as "race," and subordinate in a third set of social relations, such as in ability. The oppressed in one set of social relations can be the oppressor in another set of social relations. Thus, a person's social location and identity are complex and multiple, and simultaneously so. The relations of class, "race," gender and so on are held together and reproduced over generations by discourses or coherent knowledge systems and through cultural practices, including formal education, but also through informal processes involving the media and popular culture (McClintock 1995; Solomos and Back 1996). Discourses on gender, class and "race" fundamentally shape political economy and vice versa. These discourses have a history, having arisen in the past within a particular political economy. For instance, patriarchal gender ideologies arose in eighteenth-century England as discussed before. A variety of racist ideologies developed in the twelfth and thirteenth centuries involving the indigenous peoples of the Americas, Africa, Asia, the Middle East and others who inhabited regions that were subjected to slavery, colonialism and imperialism. These discourses are not homogenous and take on concrete forms in particular social formations and localities, in particular historical periods. As alluded to before, racism has varied from a biological discourse to a cultural discourse over time.

The nature of the issues related to racism, their inter-relationship and their articulation with other relations, such as those of class and gender, can be appreciated more clearly by examining the history of nation building in Canada.

RACISM, CLASS, GENDER AND THE "NATION" IN CANADA

The history of the development of Canada as a nation is simultaneously the history of the subjugation of Aboriginal Peoples of this continent and the deployment of immigrant groupings within its capitalist relations, as well as its articulation with racism as an ideology. A colonial, mercantile capitalism based initially on fur trading, whaling and fishing (Stevenson 1999) and later on farming and a burgeoning industrial capitalist economy was based on the appropriation of land from Aboriginal Peoples, their removal and segregation onto reserves and their extermination in some cases. The deprivation of Aboriginal communities of their land, resources and families was enabled through such laws and institutions as the *Indian Act* (first enacted in 1876) and the residential school system, to name two of the most pernicious. These laws and policies were overtly racist and patriarchal, with Aboriginal people seen as less than human and in need of civilization, which included the inculcation of Victorian patriarchal ideologies by white Christian masters who would "cleanse" them of their pre-European cultural heritages. While colonialism was being consolidated in the form of land appropriation from Aboriginal Peoples, these lands were being settled and cleared by immigrants, initially referred to as "pioneers," from England and France and later by "preferred immigrants" (white) from Western Europe and the U.S., many of whom brought along enslaved Africans. Slavery had also been prevalent in Canada since the mid-1600s, lasting up to 1833, when the British Parliament passed *The Emancipation Act*. Since 1783, there were free African American loyalists, who were invited into Canada with promises of land and a free life.

So-called "sojourners," largely men from China, India and Japan, ejected from colonial regimes of their own, were brought in around the mid-1800s to provide labour on farms, railways, mines, fisheries and factories in the new nation. These latter groups from Asia and Blacks from the U.S. were said to be "unpreferred," and every effort was made to keep them as a temporary group of migrants who would not make Canada their home. Thus, a racial hierarchy was established in the ways in which the land was dispossessed from its original inhabitants, given to white settlers, largely withheld from Asians and Black settlers, other than the worst lands in the case of Black loyalists in Nova Scotia, or confiscated, in the case of Japanese Canadians when they were classified as "enemy aliens" during World War II. While Aboriginal Peoples were segregated from and excluded from the nation build-ing process, Black and Asian workers were included but routinely subjected to racism in terms of the types of labour they could perform, the terms of their entry into Canada, their disentitlement from being full members of the nation and their tenuous status in it. I have discussed how Aboriginal Peoples and people of colour were prevented from having families of their choices (Das Gupta 2000). Initially, Aboriginal families were intentionally torn apart by the forced separation of children from their families through the militaristic residential school system (the vestiges of which lasted till 1988) and subsequently through child welfare systems. In the case of immigrants of colour, there was an intentional policy of preventing the women in those communities from settling in Canada through such systematic mechanisms as the head tax, landing fees, quotas and outright exclusionary laws. For Blacks brought as slaves, racist ideology militated against maintaining families and kin relations as family members were separated based on the whims of slave masters. Japanese families were forcibly separated during World War II and relocated in camps all over the country. In post-war times, some of these policies continued, for instance, the case of "single" domestic workers (largely Black and Asian women) and "single" farm workers (largely South American and Black men), who were prevented from bringing in their spouses and children. Other immigrants of colour faced obstacles to re-unifying their families through regulated definitions of families that were Eurocentric in nature. As in the case of Aboriginal families, nuclear and patriarchal gender relations were instituted with the help of sponsorship policies. The formula-tion of the nation as a "white nation" and Aboriginal Peoples and people of colour as outsiders in it was institutionalized through the *Indian Act* (Lawrence 2004) and through immigration laws (Jakubowski 1997). A full explication of this history is beyond this book, but the main point is that capitalist relations that developed in the nation that became known as Canada were intrinsi-cally interlocked with racism and sexism as ideologies. Those who became dominant members of the nation were white and male, and those who were excluded or marginalized were people of colour, Aboriginal people and most females, among whom white females were more privileged than their non-white counterparts. Hence, there developed an intersection of nationalism, racism, sexism and class formation in Canada.

This pattern of intersection continues. Galabuzi (2006) discusses the racialization of poverty in Canada in the late 1990s and 2000s by referring to data from Statistics Canada. He concludes that "there is a gap between the economic performance of racialized and non-racialized [white] groups when one considers such indicators as income, unemployment and labour market participation" (118).[1] He points out the particular impoverishment of racialized children, being twice that of other groups, and that of the over-sixty-five racialized group, being 13 percent above their white counterparts. He also points to the alarming poverty rates of racialized groups who live in urban centres, where newer immigrants are concentrated. Referring to other research, Galabuzi notes that the low income rate among immigrants who arrived in Canada between 1980 and 1995 varied between 47 percent in 1995 and 24.6 percent in 1980. In 2000, it stood at 35.8 percent (119). This reflects increasing levels of labour market discrimination experienced by immigrants coming into Canada between 1980 and 2000. One major feature that can account for this pattern is the fact that over this period, a larger proportion of immigrants originated in Asian, African, Caribbean, South and Central American and Middle Eastern countries, compared to earlier periods, when they originated largely from Europe and the U.S. Being mostly people of colour, these new immigrants experienced severe forms of discrimination in the labour market, which did not disappear upon settlement as in the case of earlier immigrant cohorts. These newer cohorts joined their Canadian-born racialized counterparts in the most depressed parts of the economy.

Using statistics from 2001, Galabuzi demonstrates that racialized members are over-represented in the lower-income percentiles and under-represented in the higher income percentiles. Although the median before-tax income gap between the two groups fell between 1996 and 2000, it still stood at 16.5 percent (100). A gender analysis shows that the gap was less between racialized women and non-racialized [white] women, and the former are more likely to be in clerical and sales positions, while racialized men are more likely to be among senior managers. This pattern reflects gender stereotyping and the feminization of the labour force. It also illustrates the intersection of gender and racialization and its impact on the incomes earned by women of colour. Interestingly, it indicates that gender inequalities are more significant than racial inequalities in the lives of women of colour. We will come back to this point later.

Galabuzi further shows the over-representation of racialized members in low-income occupations and sectors, most of which are non-unionized. For instance, they are over-represented in clothing and textile and banking and under-represented in the motor vehicle industry, steel industry and federal government. Galabuzi notes their particular under-representation among fire chiefs, police officers and judges. The latter fact has implications for the kind of experience people of colour have at various levels of the criminal justice system, which I explicate later in the discussion of anti-Black racism.

Overall, Galabuzi's study is an excellent demonstration of the intersection of racialization and the class structure in Canada, where those earning high incomes and in more desirable jobs are white, while those earning low incomes, many of whom are living in poverty, in non-unionized jobs, are people of colour. This pattern indicates a historical continuity of racialized social relations, which took root under colonialism and slavery several centuries back.

In a related study, Teelucksingh and Galabuzi (2005) demonstrate that the intersection between class inequalities and racialization in the Canadian labour market today is largely attributable to labour market discrimination, resulting from both racism and sexism, experienced by immigrants who entered Canada since 1990, most of whom happen to be non-white. Their research also demonstrates that there is no easy correspondence between class privilege and lack of racism. In the census period of 1996–2001, university-educated immigrants as well as those with no post-secondary education earned less, had lower levels of participation in the labour force and faced higher rates of unemployment compared to non-immigrants. As mentioned before, these realities are highly racialized and contribute to higher rates of unemployment and lower incomes of non-whites in the labour market compared to white workers despite university education. University-educated immigrants, most of whom are non-white, are systemically channelled into precarious jobs and thus low incomes through the process of devaluation of their skills and education as well as employer racism at the point of hiring. This process of devaluation is an instance of systemic racism, where the apparently neutral policies and procedures of professional and credential-giving bodies adversely affect immigrants of colour. The demand for Canadian education and experience is yet another systemic and everyday means by which employers exclude foreign educated professionals from jobs for which they are qualified. The underlying discourse tying these policies and practices together is that education in countries where these immigrants come from (e.g., Asia, Africa, South and Central America, Caribbean) is inferior. These attitudes are laced with racialized stereotypes and prejudices.

Combining immigrants and non-immigrants of colour, the income gap between white and non-white workers is larger for those without university education (particularly for those with less than high school education) and for male youth and those over sixty-five years of age. Here, we can see an intersection of racialization, class, gender and age. As far as the intersection of class and "race" are concerned, labour market discrimination, in particular racism, seems to occur among all classes of immigrants, but it seems to be at a lower degree for those with more class privilege. Racism nonetheless has a significant impact on the labour market experiences of university-educated people of colour.

While Galabuzi (2006) and Teelucksingh and Galabuzi (2005) note the importance of gender in the racialization of the labour market, they do not explicate this intersection in detail. Referring to Broad's (2000) analysis, Galabuzi notes that the current stage of capitalist development can be characterized by its "neo-liberal global economic restructuring," one of whose central features is the increased entry of women into paid work. The economy is marked by precarious jobs, including part-time, temporary, contract and own-account self employment. Precarious jobs are marked by both racialization and feminization. For a more detailed examination of the intersection of class, gender and racialization, we turn to Cranford and Vosko (2006).

Using a range of indicators to measure precarious employment,[2] Cranford and Vosko demonstrate, using statistics, that women are more represented than men in precarious forms of employment. Compared to men of colour, women of colour are less represented in full-time permanent and temporary work and more highly represented in part-time temporary and permanent work. Cranford and Vosko further point out that men of colour are more likely to be in precarious employment than white men and that there is growing convergence of the experiences of young men of colour and of women of all racialized backgrounds, thus indicating an intersection of age, gender and "race." The greatest difference in precarity seems to be between white men and women of colour thus pointing to the intersection of class, "race" and gender inequalities.

Using the indicators of unionization rate and contingency, Cranford and Vosko state that workers of colour are less unionized compared to white workers and are more likely to experience company uncertainty. However, "women of colour are the most likely to be in and out of work and to have less than a year on the job…. Differences between women along lines of race are less stark along the dimension of income and the social wage" (65–66), a fact that Galabuzi's (2006) study also alludes to.

Cranford and Vosko (2006) comment that there are differences among the category of "visible minority," the official name given to describe non-whites in Canada. These authors indicate different locations of women from different ethnicized and racialized groups depending on the indicator used to measure precarity. Hum and Simpson (2007) also warn against "hasty generalizations about the wage structure of the Canadian labour market based upon a simple comparison of non-visible and visible minorities" (91). They illustrate that while all visible minorities show lower hourly and annual earn-ings compared to non-visible minorities, there are variations in labour market characteristics of different visible minority groups, for instance, in the hourly wage, annual hours worked, etc. Ornstein's (2006) research indicates similar approaches. Existing research of labour market characteristics of various ethno-racial groups calls for more focused and precise studies of experiences in the labour market. Since the focus of this book is racism within the nursing profession and one of the largest racialized groupings among nurses is Black women, I elaborate in the next section on the ideology of anti-Black racism, its historical roots, its intersection with gender ideologies and its translation into social relations and structures in Canada.

ANTI-BLACK RACISM

Anti-Black racism[3] is an ideology directed towards individuals of African heritage and which began with the slave trade in Europe, tying together the histories of Europe, the Americas, the Caribbean and Africa. Starting in the 1400s, Portuguese sailors, with royal and papal blessings, captured Africans and sold them as house servants. Meanwhile, new trade routes were sought by both the Portuguese and the Spanish, with contacts made in India as well as South America and the Caribbean. Plantations and mining, which required large pools of labour, were forced onto the Indigenous Peoples of these regions. In the process of colonization and settlement, these people were subjected to violence, disease, destruction and death (Institute of Race Relations 1982). This is the context in which the African slave trade developed in the 1500s and continued until about 1807. The first slave landed in Quebec in 1628, and slavery continued in Canada until about 1783.

The overwhelming characteristics of the slave trade were the complete dehumanization of slaves and the sheer volume of the trade. Racist ideology developed to rationalize such mass cruelty and inhumanity. This ideology defined a Black as animal-like, less than human, having different abilities and skills and being inferior to Europeans mentally, physically, spiritually and culturally. The labour of Black men and women was seen as inferior and hence not deserving of remuneration. Moreover, there were peculiar sexual mythologies around Blacks, notions of unusually high sexual and reproduc-tive capacities, which were also connected to their so-called inhumanity and thus inferiority.

These ideologies were not only racist, but also sexist and often contradic-tory. For instance, on the one hand, Black women were portrayed as slow, de-sexed mammies, an image that evolved into the "Aunt Jemima" figure — a servile and contented Black woman cooking and serving white families. On the other hand, there was the sexual objectification of Black women's bodies (hooks 1992).

Davis (1981), Brand (1987) and Thornhill (1991) have all written on the legacies of slavery for Black women today. Thornhill writes of the stereotype of Black women as "Amazon women enduring hardships, the likes of which no 'lady' could endure" and the "tough, domineering, aggressive matriarch." Both of these stereotypes are derived from racist ideology and the fact that under slavery Black women worked in back-breaking, physical work, similar to her male counterparts. They were beaten just as harshly and dehumanized as much as Black men. They were "nullified as Women" (Thornhill 1991).

Under slavery, Black people could not maintain families on their own terms. Black women were regularly subjected to sexual violence by their masters and had to bear their children. Slave masters decided on all marriages among their slaves and frequently decided who would bear whose children. Racism as an ideology had no respect for family life among Black people. Husbands, wives, children and the elderly were separated as a normal course of events. The material and social conditions did not allow Black women to develop the attributes of upper-class, white "ladies." Their roles as mother, grandmother, daughter, worker and community builder required them to be strong and independent decision-makers and leaders.

Davis (1981) writes that since Black women were oppressed equally, if not more severely, as Black men, they resisted their oppression just as strongly. Thornhill (1991) mentions the long list of African heads of state who were female and slave leaders such as Marie-Joseph Angelique, who set fire to her mistress's house in 1734 upon discovering that she would be sold the next day. Harriet Tubman, a leader of the Underground Railroad, led over three hundred slaves out of the Southern United States into Canada. Davis writes that the resistance to slavery that women displayed was a "terrifying revelation" for slave owners, who devised "especially brute repression" to punish them, including rape. This history has given rise to the stereotypes of Black women being "aggressive," "matriarchs," "Amazons" and "dangerous." hooks (1992) writes that "radical" Black females even in modern times are often labelled "crazy" by their opponents. This is a tactic used to silence women who are outspoken in their opposition to the status quo. This tradition of organizing, leadership and outspokenness has given rise to the stereotype of Black women as "evil and treacherous."

hooks argues that the "devaluation of Black womanhood" continued beyond slavery largely as a form of social control, i.e., to prevent their accomplishments since that would destroy white supremacist ideology. Slavery-based stereotypes are kept alive in a variety of ways, for example, through the education system, most notably through the curriculum. This happens by omission and by commission. The absence of images of Black people perpetuates the impression that "they don't exist" or that "they are unimportant." Images of Black people that are included are often caricatures, portrayed in stereotypical roles, e.g., as happy helpers, manual labourers or starving victims. Language is also employed to reinforce popular stereotypes and prejudices. For instance, "blackness" is associated with danger, fear or negative things, e.g., referring to a tragic event as a "black day" or describing evil as "dark." The devil himself is sometimes portrayed as black for instance and angels as white. hooks recognizes the connection between representation and domination. In order for anti-Black racism to continue, images of Black people today reinvent and reinforce stereotypes emanating out of slavery. These images condition how non-Blacks perceive Blacks, how they interact with each other and how power is distributed along racial lines.

Even after slavery was abolished, anti-Black racism continued in the form of ideas, images and material conditions. When Black loyalists came into Canada in 1783 with promises of free land, following the American War of Independence, most were disappointed. They were served after white loyalists and either received no land or were given inferior land, with little crop potential. As a result, they ended up working as wage labourers in the homes and farms of white Canadians. Walker (1985) describes racial segregation and marginalization in residential, educational and religious lives as "caste like." The vulnerability of African Nova Scotians was driven home in the late 1960s with the bulldozing of Africville, a successful Black settlement in Halifax, for which residents remain uncompensated to this day.

The marginalization and stigmatization of Black communities continue. A number of scholarly works document the histories and geographies of Blacks in Canada (e.g., Mensah 2002). Some examples are reiterated here to illustrate the historical continuity of anti-Black racism in contemporary times. Near riot conditions prevailed on the streets of Halifax, Nova Scotia, in July 1991, involving Black youth. Similar outbursts were witnessed in Montreal and Toronto in May 1992. In these three instances, the violence indicated the disenfranchisement of Black youth from social, economic and political access within Canadian society. Unemployment among Blacks in Nova Scotia was estimated to be as high as 80 percent at the time of the disturbances.

In the aftermath of the riot in Halifax, a report (1991) written by the Nova Scotia Advisory Group on Race Relations, comprised of all three levels of government and the Black community, notes that racism is part of the daily existence of Black people in Nova Scotia:

> Black Nova Scotians still do not enjoy equal access to jobs; their businesses have difficulty succeeding because they do not have equal access to funding.... The educational system does not reflect their history and experience; the criminal justice system does not treat them fairly; they are often negatively portrayed in the media; and they cannot gain equal access to places of entertainment such as bars.

A more recent study (Mensah 2002: 91) notes a similar reality. Using statistics from 1999, Mensah asserts that Blacks in Nova Scotia are over-represented among people with grade nine level education and "acutely under-represented" among those with bachelor's or higher degrees. Moreover, they are over-represented in low-level jobs, such as in sales and service and semi-skilled manual work, and experience a 20 percent rate of unemployment, higher than that experienced by other visible minorities and by all Nova Scotians. Mensah adds that "a quarter of Blacks [in Nova Scotia] have annual incomes of under $5,000" (92).

Another report, which is pointed in its discussion of anti-Black racism (Lewis 1992), was written in the aftermath of the May 1992 "Yonge Street riots" in Toronto. Lewis pointed out that it is the Black community that is shot at by police, streamed in schools, forced to "drop out," subjected to racism in Metro Toronto Housing Authority's subsidized housing facilities and denied employment equity. He mentioned that many members of the Black community, particularly parents, live in fear of encounters with the police. This is because of frequent shootings of Black youth by police.

One recommendation of the Lewis Report led to the establishment of the Royal Commission on Race Relations in the Criminal Justice System. The Commission's report (1994) confirmed anti-Black racism, particularly in prison environments. Overtly racist language, harassment and excessive force against Black prisoners were said to be common practices. Stereotypes of Black men and women reminiscent of slavery were dominant, with a senior administrator reporting that "Black people are feared, considered dangerous."

Based on these reports and theorizing about anti-Black racism, a number of landmark decisions were made in Ontario courts. In a Court of Appeal decision (1992) involving Carlton Parks, a Black male convicted of manslaughter of a white male, Justice David Doherty discussed the reality of anti-Black racism in Canada and in particular in Metro Toronto:

> I do not pretend to essay a detailed critical analysis… however, I must accept the broad conclusions repeatedly expressed in these materials. Racism, and in particular anti-Black racism, is a part of our community psyche. A significant segment of our community holds overtly racist views. A much larger segment subconsciously operates on the basis of negative racial stereotypes. (29)

Justice Doherty ruled that the conviction of the Black male was to be quashed because his lawyer had been prevented by the trial judge from asking potential jurors about their ability to be impartial, given that the accused is Black and the victim is white.

In 1996, in *Regina v. Wilson* (1996), there was an appeal of the decision of a trial judge to disallow challenging prospective jurors on the basis of anti-Black racism following from Justice Doherty's ruling. The trial judge had claimed that anti-Black racism existed in Metropolitan Toronto and not elsewhere. The case involved a Black man, allegedly a drug dealer in Whitby, Ontario. There had been no violence or white victim as in the Carlton Parks case. The appeal was granted on the basis that anti-Black racism does not stop at the border of Metropolitan Toronto.

In a more controversial case, *Regina v. R.D.S* (1995), Judge Corinne Sparks, who happens to be the first African Canadian judge in Nova Scotia and the first African Canadian female judge in Canada, issued a ruling in the trial of a fifteen-year-old Black youth who had been arrested by a white police officer for resisting the arrest of his cousin. She ruled in favour of the youth, referring to police racism, particularly anti-Black racism. Her ruling was appealed by the Crown and Judge Sparks was found to be biased against the white police officer. A new trial was ordered, although there was a dissenting opinion by Judge Freeman.[4] What amounted to the disciplining and silencing of Judge Sparks shows continuing anti-Black racism in the criminal justice system, in this case in Nova Scotia.

What Judge Sparks had been referring to was anti-Black racism in the police force, which leads to the over-policing of Black youths, which in turn leads to over-representation of Black youths among those charged and arrested. A *Toronto Star* (2002a) story highlighted the problem of racial profiling[5] by police officers, a problem that had been pointed out by members of the Black community for decades. Toronto police traffic offence data obtained by the *Star* revealed that "a disproportionate number of Blacks have been ticketed for violations that routinely surface only after a traffic stop has been made." Although Blacks made up only 8.1 percent of the city's population, 34 percent of drivers charged were Black. In some patrol areas, over 50 percent of those charged were Black. In contrast, 52.1 percent of those charged were white even though 62.7 percent of the city's population was white. Moreover, Blacks were over-represented in the arrest statistics. Most of those charged were men between the ages of twenty-five and thirty-four. Many members of the Black community and academics argue that the statistics reveal over-policing in the Black community, an institutional practice based on the stereotype that Black males were more prone to criminality, a stereotype emanating from the history of slavery and post-slavery periods. Racial profiling among police is an excellent example of a racial formation, a concept developed by Omi and Winant (1994), discussed earlier, which connects representational and ideological aspects of racism with structural aspects. However, just as Judge Sparks was silenced in the case of *Regina v. R.D.S (1995)*, similarly there was denial from Police Chief Fantino that racism had anything to do with the statistics. In another story in the same series, the *Star* (2002b) revealed differential and harsher treatment given to Blacks charged with drug possession compared to whites. Blacks were released less often at the scene compared to whites and they were jailed more often while waiting for a bail hearing.

The *Star's* series on racial profiling sparked a debate on the collection of race-based statistics. While the Police Services Board has a strict policy of not publicizing or analyzing "race"-based data recorded internally, some advocated the maintenance and analysis of such data to fight racism in policing. Others advocated against it or keeping only partial data to document differential treatment without stigmatizing any racialized community. The "everyday" nature of racial profiling was apparent at a hearing called by the Ontario Human Rights Commission (Keung and Hutsul 2003) following the *Star* series. Some eight hundred people responded to the chief commissioner's call for incident reports of racial profiling. In 2007, an Ontario Human Rights Commission tribunal declared racial profiling as a violation of the Ontario Human Rights Code in the case of a Black woman who was accused of shoplifting a $10 item in a mall, repeatedly searched and subjected to verbal abuse, just because she was Black and perceived to being a "foreigner" and "not speaking English." The incident happened in 2003, at the end of which she was released without charge. This incident revealed not only the racialization of crime, racial profiling and racist policing, it also revealed a classist racialization of the nation as a whole where a working-class Black woman was assumed to be a "foreigner," a non-Canadian, an outsider to the nation and subjected to coercion and denied human rights as a result.

The media articles and Commission report corroborated what criminologist Wortley and Tanner (2003) argued all along through their research. After statistically controlling for a variety of factors (criminal activity, drug use, gang membership, etc.), which could also influence stop and search statistics, Wortley and Tanner demonstrated through a survey of 3,393 high school students that Black students are much more likely to be stopped and searched by police than white, Asian and other racialized students. Moreover, they illustrated that variations in age, social class and "being on good behaviour" do not prevent Black youths from being stopped and searched by police.

Following these revelations, a Superior Court of Justice judge threw out a case against a Black man who had been stopped, searched and charged with drug possession by two Toronto police officers. The judge ruled that the only reason why the man was stopped and searched was that he was "a Black man with an expensive car" (Small 2004). The common-sensical assumption often is that a Black man cannot legitimately own an expensive car; he must have stolen it. Again, it is the assumption of the criminality of a Black man, a historically derived stereotype, a part of anti-Black racism. This phenomenon is now referred to as "driving while Black." Earlier, in

2001, another case against a Black man, who had been stopped near the Eaton Centre in Toronto and charged with a drug offence, was thrown out due to the use of racial profiling. This time, the accused was on foot. It is increasingly becoming clear that racial profiling and anti-Black racism are not just confined to Toronto — it has also been identified in Montreal (Cernetig 2005), in addition to Nova Scotia, as discussed earlier. Chances are that it is a national phenomenon.

Labour market research continues to suggest that Black men and women are at a disadvantage. Utilizing 2001 census data in the Toronto Census Metro Area (CMA), Ornstein (2006) concludes that "extreme economic disadvantage is highly racialized. All twenty of the poorest ethno-racial groups in the Toronto CMA are non-European" (v–vi), with the following ethno-racial groups experiencing extreme disadvantage: Grenadians, Somalians, Jamaicans, other Caribbeans, Black and multiple Caribbeans. The average unemployment rate for African (not including Caribbean) men exceeded 10 percent compared to less than 5 percent for Europeans.

Human capital differences, such as education, age and length of residence in Canada, may have an effect on labour market characteristics. However, even after adjusting for these factors, African men are still worse off, earning 25 percent less than European men. The income gap is slightly lower for African women at 17 percent. Corroborating Galabuzi (2006) and Cranford and Vosko (2006), Ornstein notes that the difference in average income of women and men in the same ethno-racial group is larger than income differences between men or women from different ethno-racial groups. Nonetheless, it is evident that Black women and other women of colour experience both racism vis-à-vis white European women and sexism vis-à-vis Black men, although sexism seems to have more impact in terms of income disadvantage.

Compared to the 10 percent poverty rate experienced by European groups, 22 percent of Caribbeans, 35 percent of Blacks and 40 percent of Africans experience poverty in Toronto CMA. More than 50 percent of Somalians experience poverty. It is noteworthy that for Caribbean groups, poorer labour market outcomes persist despite higher labour force participation rates. Ornstein notes that the poverty rate for Blacks is higher in Montreal and lower in Vancouver than in the Toronto CMA. The latter pattern was also pointed out by Mensah (2002).

Hum and Simpson (2007) illustrate statistically that overall racial status has no impact on the wage rates of native-born men and women. However, immigrant status does have an adverse effect on the wage rates of men of colour suggesting that immigration status is more significant than "race" in determining one's wages, although it has no significant effect for women of colour. The situation is different for Black men, who experience a 22 percent wage gap with their white counterparts, both for those who are immigrant and those who are born in Canada. This suggests that it is Black men's racialization that affects their wage disadvantage rather than their immigration status.[6] Hum and Simpson point out that this pattern has persisted in studies conducted in 1971, 1981, 1986, 1991 and 1999.

So far, the discussion in this chapter has been on debates around "race," racism, anti-Black racism and their articulations with nation-building, gender and class in the context of Canada. In the rest of the chapter, I link this discussion to an examination of how these concepts and historical realities play out in local institutional sites, particularly in paid workplaces. In this section, I refer to insights gathered by the Ontario Human Rights Commission,[7] which has had to grapple with the new face of racism in the province. As a result, Commission statements provide some of the best discussions of racial harassment.

RACISM IN PAID WORKPLACES TODAY

As critical race scholars have noted, new discourses of "race" stay away from the use of "race as biology," which was prevalent in earlier years. Racism in paid workplaces is also disguised, thus making it challenging to identify, understand and combat. For example, racism is hidden in management-staff conflicts over issues of competence. There are at least two reasons for the difficulty in naming racial harassment in the workplace today. First, as alluded to before, there is no apparent discourse of "race" associated with acts of everyday racism in the workplace. Second, each individual racist action or word experienced by complainants is small and appears to be trivial.

It can be difficult to name racial harassment when there is no articulation by the perpetrator of singling out a worker because of her ethnicity, racial status or colour. The harassing incidents are not associated with a racial comment, slur or joke. In fact, when charged, the perpetrator's reaction is to immediately and vociferously deny the harassment and the racism. Typically, higher management in workplaces (hospitals) join the immediate manager in denying that any harassment took place.

While the Ontario Human Rights Commission includes under racial harassment such acts as slurs and jokes, ridicules, insults or name calling on the basis of race, colour, ancestry, religion, ethnicity, citizenship or language (OHRC 2001), it recognizes that it also includes "any vexatious comment or conduct that is known or ought reasonably to be known to be unwelcome." This implies that the individual being harassed does not always have to explicitly object to harassing behaviour. The OHRC (2001) recognizes that a person in a vulnerable position may not be able to object to harassment from someone in a position of power.

The Ontario Human Rights Commission further expounds on the different facets of harassment. For instance, it states that harassing incidents may be racist even when they are not directed towards a person of colour or a minority person. Harassing behaviour violates the rights of the person who is the subject of the comment as well as the person privy to the behaviour, whether that person is a person of colour, of a minority group from a different racialized group or a white person who associates with a racialized person. If such behaviours — racist jokes, cartoons or pictures — are generally present in a workplace, they create a "poisoned environment," which hurts and makes people of colour and minority people uncomfortable, thereby denying them equality. Harassment does not have to be continuous in order to create a poisoned environment; it could be a single incident or comment that creates discomfort.

The Ontario Human Rights Commission (2001) recognizes that comments or conduct do not have to be explicit to constitute racial harassment, i.e., that it may result from differential treatment, such as being arbitrarily disciplined and monitored. In recognizing this point, the OHRC acknowledges that in today's society, racism in action may not always be accompanied with the language of "race," as the latter is incongruent with state-sanctioned policies, laws and even cultural practices, given decades of community struggle for human rights and equity, at local, national and international levels.

Racial harassment can be overt or subtle. When it is overt, such as in the form of name-calling, a direct joke or outright violence, it is easy to identify. Racial harassment that is indirect or covert is difficult to identify, as illustrated by Joan's story in the introduction to this book.

Racial harassment of the type that Joan experienced is common in today's workplaces. Legislation and workplace policies and procedures are often invoked by management to counsel or discipline non-white workers, ultimately resulting in their resignation or dismissal, while the same laws, policies and procedures are often not applied as rigorously for white workers. As I have argued before (Das Gupta 1996a), white workers and workers of colour are "managed" differently because they are seen to be fundamentally different due to their "race."

In addition to critical race theories and the "race, gender and class" approach as discussed in preceding sections, I draw from critical political economy traditions within sociology, particularly from a feminist perspective. Bringing all these diverse paradigms together, I refer to my approach as Marxist, feminist and anti-racist (Das Gupta 1996a). In the following section, I discuss feminist literature from a Marxist political economy perspective because a discussion of women's work, both paid and unpaid, is the larger context within which the work of nursing should be viewed.

MARXIST FEMINIST POLITICAL ECONOMY

In Marxist, neo-Marxist and traditional political economy writings (Bottomore 1983: 375), the formal economy and paid workplaces, most notably factories, workshops and other sites where workers sell their labour power, are the focus of research. In formal workplaces those who own or control the means of production (the bourgeoisie) and those who do not (the proletariat) enter into social relations and fight a class struggle over wages, the labour process, conditions of work, benefits, health and safety issues, autonomy, etc. Until recently, this was implicitly and explicitly assumed to be a male dominated world, where women's incursions were seen as anomalous and deviant. Marx (1967: 394) discussed women workers as "supplementary labour power," drawn on with the advent of machinery in capitalist workplaces. As industrialization deepened, women workers were utilized when the need arose and then expelled when the need no longer existed. This was demonstrated perhaps most clearly during and after World War II, when women were asked to take on male defined work because most of the menfolk were in the military. Once the war was over, women were asked to go back to their homes and sacrifice their jobs for the returning men (Vosko 2000: 88). In Western European-based societies, including Canada, as industrialization developed and the market economy came into being in the eighteenth century onwards, a spatial separation developed between waged work and unwaged household and caregiving work. There was simultaneously an ideological shift, with women's main sphere of operation seen as the "private" domestic realm. It is based on this ideological separation of men's and women's spheres of paid and unpaid work that current notions of gender emerged. Within this scenario Marx's notion of women being utilized within capitalism as a reserve army of labour becomes comprehensible. McClintock (1995: 168) writes "the cult of industrial rationality and the cult of domesticity formed a crucial but concealed alliance." Thus, with the identification of women within the private, domestic sphere, women in our society began to be associated with caregiving, nurturing, cooking, cleaning, mending, assisting and teaching, while men began to be associated with providing leadership and being physically strong and active in the public world. It must be noted though that this was a classed and racialized process. McClintock (1995: 160) writes that the ideal of middle-class womanhood was to be "idle" and a "lady of leisure." The work that she performed (even with the help of women and men servants) was to be invisible. She became simply ornamental. McClintock (1995) writes that a working-class woman (presumably white, but having associations of "Blackness") was represented as scrubbing dirt, hauling coal from mines, serving and looking after middle-upper-class children and similar occupations. She makes an important note that there was a discrepancy between the representation of upper-middle-class Victorian (white) women in general as ladies of leisure and the lived realities of women in the middle-classes, most of whom could not afford many servants. Most wives worked hard at home in caregiving and keeping an immaculate home, but they had the added function of making sure their labour was invisible. The hegemonic and thus desirable images of the "idle (white) domestic woman" and "active (white) economic man" were born. I would add that for upper-class (mainly white) women, helpers, servants and caregivers have been women and men of colour. When slavery flourished, they were frequently Black women and men and some working-class white women. Servants were also Asian and Aboriginal women (in the North American context). McClintock writes that when poor white women worked as servants, they were often racialized as non-white. Historically, therefore, there was a discrepancy between the hegemonic ideological (white, European) notions of masculinity and femininity and the actual lived realities of women and men of colour, of poor white women and some middle-class women as well.

Gender ideologies originating in Victorian England are still with us today, albeit with variations. What has changed though is that women across racial lines are no longer a reserve army of labour. Their paid labour is now an integral part of the mainstream of capitalist labour processes. Nonetheless, ideologies born within Victorian England continue to be transmitted in the labour market, where we find most women still concentrated in sales, retail, clerical and health-related occupations (Statistics Canada 2000). The archetypical paid work for women of all time is paid domestic work, which frequently does not appear in official statistics, thus maintaining its discursive position as "non-work." Today, this work is predominantly performed in upper-class urban homes (including the homes of some upper-class families of colour) by Black, Asian and South and Central American women, generally women of colour. Not only is women's labour still seen to be more suited to occupations associated with their reproductive roles within households, it is also seen as unskilled and inferior, labour that springs from nature, that does not require training or a formal learning process. The process of learning reproductive labour through gendered socialization processes are not acknowledged in this discourse as gender itself is viewed as a biological fact. It can be argued that any occupation based on domestic roles has the stigma of "non-work" because of the historical association with the Victorian (white) middle-class "lady of leisure." (White) men's labour in contrast is seen as skilled and superior because it is subject to education and long periods of training in formal settings. It is considered "real" work, again a holdover from the Victorian image of the "economic (white) man." As alluded to before, more and more women (white and non-white), including ones with pre-school children, are part of the paid labour force (Statistics Canada 2000). They have even entered areas that were previously considered white male spheres, such as medicine and supervisory occupations. However, it is questionable whether this changing reality has challenged hegemonic patriarchal ideologies around divisions of labour. Statistical studies reveal that women (be they unpaid "wives" or paid housekeepers and caregivers of colour) still perform the bulk of housework and caregiving work in our society, despite fulfilling a larger share of paid work. Patriarchal ideologies are so powerful that they can adapt to changing realities. For instance, when women enter occupations that are non-traditional for them, often the wages and working conditions in those occupations become lowered to "suit" their socially subordinate status. This has been noted in the legal field (Rosenberg et al. 2002: 250) and in clerical work, with increasing numbers of women recruited into it over the twentieth century (Hamilton 1996: 158). This is part of the phenomenon of the feminization of labour, which many feminist authors have discussed (Vosko 2000: 34). The call for pay equity has been one policy measure to address discrimination in pay for women, not only for similar or the same work done by men, but also for different work of equal value (Hamilton 1996: 160).

FEMINIST POLITICAL ECONOMY

Smith (1992) critiqued the apparent fixation with the world of paid work and the invisibility of "household work and of childrearing" (11) as representing the "standpoint of the 'relations and apparatus of ruling'" (9), which marginalizes women's experiences. As a result, even progressive political economy becomes textualized, a discourse divorced from actual lived relations of individual men and women with racial, ethnic, age and other differences.

Feminists (Armstrong and Armstrong 1996; 1990; Connelly and Armstrong 1992) have developed the notion that the household, the unpaid work within it and gender relations are integral aspects of political economy, with production relations in the world of paid work intrinsically connected to reproductive work, i.e., in the household, the realm of unpaid work. In fact, they are not two mutually exclusive spheres. The connection between waged labour and unpaid domestic labour referred to as "reproductive labour" or as "social reproduction (the daily and generational maintenance of the labour supply)"(Vosko 2000: 39), has been a source of significant debate among Canadian feminists (Armstrong and Armstrong 1990: 67). The participants in the "domestic labour debate" theorize that women's role within social reproduction influences the gendered division of labour within waged work, conditions the relationship between men and women, and influences their identities. Moreover, the organization of domestic labour and the organization of the household are influenced by the nature of the waged labour market and one's location within class relations. Policymakers seem to be cognizant of these relationships as, when they enact new policies, they frequently do so with households and unpaid labour in mind, although they may not admit it.

For example, when cutbacks were made to institutionalized healthcare through privatization in Ontario (Armstrong et al. 2001), there was an assumption that caring work would be picked up by precarious workers, including part-time, temporary and contract workers (many of whom are women of colour and immigrant women), and by unpaid workers, who are mainly women.

This chapter describes some of the debates in the theorizing of "race," racism, gender, class and related issues. It throws light on racism in Canada, with an emphasis on the economic sphere and particular reference to African/Black Canadians. It looks at the intersectional nature of social relations, including those involving racialization, class and gender. The discussion in this chapter provides a foundation for the next chapter, on the dynamics of healthcare infrastructure, within which the work of nursing is located.

NOTES

1. Galabuzi uses the term "racialized groups" to refer to "non-Aboriginal people of colour" (xvi). This usage is different from the way in which I have utilized the concept of "racialization." I prefer to use the terms "people of colour" and "white" as I view all groups as being racialized in different ways. However, in discussing Galabuzi's work, I will stick to his terminology. Needless to say, the issue of naming racial categories is a problematic affair, one that can be the subject of a separate study.

2. The indicators include form of employment, earnings, social wage, regulatory protection and control, social location and occupational context (Cranford and Vosko, 2006: 52).

3. A large portion of this section is taken from Tania Das Gupta, *Racism and Paid Work* (Toronto: Garamond Press) 1996, p. 16 ff.

4. For a detailed analysis of this case, see Devlin, n.d.

5. Racial profiling is defined by the Ontario Human Rights Commission as "any action undertaken for reasons of safety, security or public protection that relies on stereotypes about race, colour, ethnicity, ancestry, religion, or place of origin rather than on reasonable suspicion, to single out an individual for greater scrutiny or different treatment (Ontario Human Rights Commission 2005).

6. The situation seems to be somewhat similar for native-born Latin-American men, who experience a wage gap of 38.8 percent with their white counterparts, even higher than that for Black men.

7. Ontario Human Rights Commission, *Policy and Guidelines on Racism and Racial Discrimination*, June 9, 2005. <http://www.ohrc-on.ca>

3. THE POLITICAL ECONOMY OF HEALTHCARE

This chapter discusses healthcare as a site of paid work. I present some of its key characteristics and discuss the nature of women's work in it, in particular the work of women of colour. I also provide a larger, somewhat historical, context within which contemporary experiences of nurses can be viewed. One can clearly see continuities in terms of the persistence of racism, sexism and class inequalities in this sector, specifically the reality of anti-Black racism. The chapter ends with a discussion of the research methods I used to gather information on contemporary experiences of racism in nursing in the province of Ontario.

GENDER, CLASS AND HEALTHCARE

The division of labour within healthcare is highly gendered. Doctors and administrators are predominantly male, while nurses and patients are predominantly female. It is not a coincidence that nurses are a highly feminized workforce as their caregiving role is an extension of the historical roles that women have played as unpaid caregivers in households and societies at large. Indeed, much of the work in the healthcare system is an extension of women's unpaid work traditionally performed in the home or within neighbourhoods, including cleaning, cooking and volunteer work. Moreover, within healthcare, nurses have always been subordinate to doctors, who are predominantly male.

Gendered discourses in healthcare in contemporary times need to be understood within the larger context of political and economic shifts in Canada. Such a perspective reveals the inter-class elements within nursing as an occupation as well as their intersections with gender and race discourses. Armstrong et al. (2001), Grinspun (2000) and Campbell (1988) describe the post-1970s neo-liberal paradigm shift internationally and within Canada, which steered healthcare towards a market-driven, corporatized system, where private sector strategies were implemented to supposedly rectify the alleged wasteful and inefficient public sector, in which the healthcare sector has been located in the post-war period. It was implied (Armstrong et al. 2001: 19) that women, as the majority of healthcare users as well as employees, had been abusing the system by taking state-funded universal healthcare for granted and not being responsible about it. The level of unionization was relatively high in the public sector and women benefited from that, being the majority of healthcare workers. Critics of the welfare state argued that the inefficiency and wastefulness of the public sector had contributed to a huge debt, which the state now had to pay off. This was to be done by cutting back public services and reverting to privatization, competition and creating partnerships between the private and public sectors. Strategies of cost reduction included contracting out services, adopting management techniques from the private sector, implementing user-fees, reducing unionized staff through lay-offs and substituting with non-unionized precarious workers, reducing hospital stays and transferring care to unpaid caregivers in the community, who everyone knows are mostly women. Thus, the new paradigm affected women negatively as patients and as healthcare workers.

THE DESKILLING OF MIDDLE-CLASS PROFESSIONALS

The group of women workers being looked at in this book, i.e., nurses, is often not seen as part of the working classes. This could be derivative of the notion that women workers are "not real workers." Within such a mindset, women's caregiving work, even when it is waged, is seen to be either a "labour of love" or aimed at earning "pin money." It has an association with middle-class women's domestic role, which has a historical connection with such discourses as the "cult of domesticity" and "ladies of leisure" prominent in Victorian England. As discussed before, middle-class women had to perform all the labour within the home, but make it appear as if they were idle. This was a "class" act as well since most working-class wives were unable to fulfil such an image.

Nurses are thought of as a middle-class, professional group of women, having high levels of education, earning good incomes and being unionized, thus enjoying a fairly high level of job security. Nursing has a reputation of being one of the best professions for women in the post-war period. It allows professional autonomy, flexibility and an independence that is rare. Women involved in this profession are seen as middle class compared to their sisters in clerical, sales and domestic work.

What is not readily apparent is that there are different categories of nurses, each of which requires different levels of education and experience and commands different levels of income, skill and autonomy. Thus, not all nurses are in the middle class. For instance, registered nurses (RNs) work directly with patients in delivering healthcare. Those who assist nurses include registered practical nurses (RPNs) and nurses' aides. Some RNs work in management or administration. Thus, nursing is a highly segmented and hierarchical profession. Each of the rungs of the hierarchy has a different level of income, autonomy and location within authority structures. Thus, it appears that just as in Victorian middle-class households, where the housewife was expected to maintain an air of leisure with the help of servants, similarly in nursing, registered nurses, especially those in supervisory positions, are expected to maintain an atmosphere in which they have the added responsibility of erasing any signs of work (McClintock 1995: 162) with the help of layers of nurse assistants.

Since the 1990s, there has been a dramatic shift in the perception of nursing based on their increasing proletarianization. Some nurses have left their profession, some have left Canada to practise elsewhere and many others have spoken out about the worsening conditions within hospitals and healthcare in general, which have impacted negatively on their working conditions. This is a reflection of funding cutbacks initiated by the federal government under the Canada Health and Social Transfer program and the restructuring of healthcare overall, which set up a number of dynamics that fundamentally restructured the work of nursing and transformed the image of nurses as a well-off, middle-class group of professionals. Nursing, which had always been a segmented workforce, has now become further segmented with growing levels of deskilling and degradation, features usually associated with the working classes. Campbell (1988) notes that, in the name of "quality assurance," nurses are being monitored more through "form filing." Scientific management principles are being deployed in hospitals without any thought to the impact on patient care, let alone relations among employees.

These trends were well recognized by nurses in the 1980s. A survey (Murray and Smith 1988) of 1,240 registered nurses in Metro Toronto revealed that most were feeling negative about nursing as a career and would not recommend it to others. About 15–30 percent were contemplating leaving their jobs.[1] Responses to the survey suggested that nurses were dissatisfied with their pay as well as their inability to use their skills. Nurses' comments implied that "broadening of pay ranges based on experience and expertise," a "reduction in non-nursing duties" and "more patient contact" would increase their level of satisfaction. Sixty percent of nurses reported conflicts with physicians, and about half said that they never got support from nursing administration when they were in such situations. Eighty-six percent reported "some" or "a lot" of stress related to working conditions, job politics, lack of respect and patient care issues.

A review of twenty-one provincial studies between 1987 and 1989 conducted by the Canadian Nurses' Association (CNA) and the Canadian Hospital Association (CHA) (1990) summarized the problems of nurses who had subsequently opted out of the workforce. The responsibility for this trend lay in poor working conditions, including inadequate staffing to ensure quality of patient care, inflexible work schedules, increases in non-nursing duties, lack of professional autonomy, lack of participation in decision-making and lack of collegial respect.

This was the nursing context in Ontario in 1994, when the *Regulated Health Professions Act* (RHPA) ushered in contradictory dynamics for nurses, a predominantly female workforce. On the one hand, the Act recognized nurses as a professional group, rather than handmaidens of a male-dominated medical workforce (Lum and Williams 2000), allowing them to regulate their own profession through the College of Nurses of Ontario. It also recognized nurse practitioners as independent primary caregivers. On the other hand, the Act allowed for the utilization of unregulated care providers (UCPs) who only receive a few weeks to few months of training and are lower paid than RNs, wherever feasible.

In Canada, the acceptance of UCPs indicated greater de-skilling and thus fragmentation among nurses themselves. It allowed administrations to cut costs by replacing RNs and RPNs in certain areas with UCPs, thus increasing the proportion of contingent and cheapened labour. While full-time RNs decreased from 45,360 in 1994 to 41,064 in 1999, part-timers increased from 35,941 to 37,133 (CIHI [Canadian Institute for Health Information] 2000). The latter trend included underemployment, where RNs and RPNs were working in positions where UCPs worked. The employment of UCPs has raised concerns around the quality of care and safety of patients. In addition, since UCPs are supervised by RNs or RPNs, any nursing errors committed by UCPs are attributed to their supervisors. Needless to say, this puts additional pressure on RNs and RPNs.

The unemployment rate among nurses in Canada had risen as well. Between 1994 and 1999, RNs employed in nursing declined from 81,301 to 78,197 (CIHI 2000). The Health Sector Training and Adjustment Program (HSTAP) reported that almost 21,000 health employees were laid off or faced casualization between 1994 and 1997. Most of these were in the hospital sector, while the numbers of registered nurses employed in community health centres increased from 1994 to 1997. Registered nurses in community health centres, which includes public health units, community care access centres and homecare services, generally earn 5 to 20 percent lower salaries compared to those working in hospitals.[2] Salary increases are generally not more then 2 percent per year due to funding limitations of community health centres. In addition, pay equity adjustments in this sector during the 1990s were hampered by restrictions imposed by the Harris government, including abolishment of the proxy comparison method[3] and funding cap in 1996 (ONA 1997). Although the proxy method was reinstated in 1997 following a successful Charter challenge by Service Employees International Union, Local 204, and two women, the government only paid retroactive proxy pay equity funding for 1995–97. Since then, no additional funding has been allocated by the government for sectors in which the proxy method has to be used, including community health sectors.[4]

RACE, GENDER AND CLASS IN HEALTHCARE

My research is based within an anti-racist feminist political economy approach of healthcare, which goes beyond simply looking at gender issues. Moreover, I begin from the experiences of nurses of colour and locate them within the larger political economy of healthcare. Historically derived race, gender and class discourses impact on this political economy reflecting both old and new ideas around women of colour and immigrant women in paid workplaces. Within the gendered labour force in healthcare, observations and studies have confirmed that women of colour are by and large located in the lower levels of the system, in the most precarious sectors. This is a reflection of a racialized gender structure, where women of colour are assigned to cleaning, cooking and assisting white women with their caregiving work. Critiquing feminist analysis, Nestel (2000) argues that healthcare does not reflect the gendered division of labour in traditional households but rather reflects that in "newly reconstituted bourgeoise families," where caring work is done by immigrant women and women of colour, leaving the (white) woman of the house to engage in professional labour. Just as in Victorian English upper-middle-class homes, where white women maintained a cult of domesticity with the help of female servants, so also nursing managers and administrators, predominantly white, maintain a cult of domesticity in hospital wards with the help of registered nurses, registered practical nurses, nursing assistants and aides, who have significant concentrations of women of colour among them. Within Western capitalist political economies, even in their subordinate position as women, white women historically enjoyed certain privileges as "mothers of the nation" (Dua 1999). In contrast, women of colour were seen historically as "threats" to the nation, with their reproductive powers and sexuality seen as challenging its whiteness. In addition, women of colour and immigrant women were seen as inferior in their reproductive roles to white women. Maternal feminists in the first wave devoted considerable time to "civilizing" and "teaching" proper womanly skills to such subordinated groups of women. This mindset has lasted through the ages and is reflected in paid workplaces even today.

Many precariously employed caregivers are immigrant women and women of colour (Vosko 2000; de Wolff 2000) who are new in Canada, trying to establish themselves here and trying to continue with or enter one of the caring professions, for example, nursing. Rosen (2001) of the Filipino Nurses Support Group writes that thousands of educated and skilled Filipino nurses have been recruited into Canada under the Live-in Caregiver Program (LICP) to work as nannies and home support workers. They could not qualify under the points system because nurses were not in demand. In addition, these nurses faced problems in getting their qualifications recognized and were thus forced to work for low wages for private agencies catering to wealthy clients, who were mainly white. According to Rosen, they were paid one-third the wages made by registered nurses, some as low as $700 per month. Presently, their bargaining strength is curtailed by the fact that they are contractually required to live with and provide nursing or care to a Canadian family for two years before they can apply for immigration status. As alluded to before, one can argue that the devaluation of the professional qualifications and experiences of immigrant nurses of colour and their consequent underemployment and low remuneration are discourses of racialization that see "immigrant," read non-white outsiders, to the Nation of Canada, as inferior to the hegemonic whiteness characterizing the latter. Such practices occur as a result of racist discourses that assume that non-whites or members of the Global South possess inferior education and experiences compared to those available in Canada. A devaluation of regions of the world becomes extended into a devaluation of the people coming from those regions. Moreover, in a pre-dominantly women's occupation that is highly racially structured, non-white immigrant women nurses are assumed to be inferior in relation to their white, Canadian counterparts.

Racialized labour supplies have been historically regulated by profes-sional bodies such as the College of Nurses, nurse training institutions and the state through its immigration and sponsorship rules and special schemes, such as the Live-in Caregiver Program. Calliste (1993) writes that Canadian nursing schools did not admit Canadian-born Black students before the 1940s on the pretext that hospitals would not employ them. This policy was challenged successfully by the Nova Scotia Association for the Advancement of Coloured People, supported by some unions and churches. Between 1950 and 1962, Canadian immigration authorities started to admit limited numbers of Caribbean nurses in response to the urgings of groups like the Negro Citizenship Association. However, they were admitted under rules quite different from those governing the entry of white nurse immigrants. Calliste argues that Black nurses were required to have nursing qualifications "over and above" those required for White nurses.

Gustafson (2002) notes that, although a few Japanese and Chinese Canadian women were admitted to the Vancouver General Hospital Training School in the 1930s, upon graduation they could only practise within their own communities. She reports that, during the World War II period, with its shifting attitudes regarding women's work, increasing stratification among groups of nurses and demands for nursing labour, space opened up for nurses of colour to be incorporated into the mainstream.

Hine (1989) documents the history of exclusion of African-American women from U.S. schools and hospitals responsible for training nurses in the late nineteenth century. She notes that training schools in the northern U.S. operated with racial quotas, while those in the south completely denied admission to Black candidates, who were also excluded from the American Nurses' Association. The African-American community had to establish its own schools and associations, and some Canadian Black women aspiring to be nurses attended these schools as a result of racial exclusion in Canadian institutions.

Lack of access to nursing training experienced by people of colour in the U.S in more recent times, particularly at university levels, is noted as a concern by McCloskey and Grace (1997) and by the Minority Nurse Editors (2001). While 11 percent of Americans are Black, only 4.9 percent of nurses are Black. It is noteworthy that a higher proportion of Black nurses held master's and doctoral degrees compared to non-Black nurses. Spanish-speaking peoples constitute 8.6 percent of American population, yet only 2 percent of nurses are Spanish-speaking. Only Asians, at 3 percent of U.S. population, are reflected proportionately in nursing, at 3.7 percent (Minority Nurse Editors 2001).

Lee-Cunin (1989) documents the lack of access to nursing schools in Britain. Carlisle (1990) writes about the disincentives for young people of colour to entering nursing, including required English levels and marginalization in training due to the Eurocentric curriculum.

After overcoming the hurdles of training, licensing and being hired in their profession, many nurses of colour face marginalization and discriminatory treatment. Head (1985) notes that in 1983 a group of about a hundred ethnic minority nurses and healthcare workers in Toronto came together over experiences of workplace racism, including segregation in the least desirable levels of the nursing hierarchy and lack of promotional prospects. The group was known as The Healthcare Team. They alleged that a disproportionate number of nurses of colour were subjected to discipline due to minor nursing errors and reported to the College of Nurses for breaches of nursing standards. Many such complaints, often not investigated thoroughly, led to dismissals and suspensions of nursing licenses. It was also alleged by members of The Team that some nurses of colour had been disciplined for expressing disagreement with their supervisors, while white nurses had not been treated in the same manner.

GENDER AND RACE ISSUES IN THE NURSING CRISIS

Studies show that racism, particularly overt forms, increases during economic crises and falls during boom periods (Muszynski and Reitz 1982; OFL 1981; Head 1985). A U.K. study (Winkelmann-Gleed 2007) shows that restructuring and the associated implementation of new public management approaches in the National health Service have resulted in increased discrimination faced by Black and minority ethnic (BME) nurses. The author demonstrates that the discrimination has been exacerbated in a context of "uncertainty and pressure in form of workload, staffing and finances caused by organizational restructuring" (18). Winkelmann-Gleed further suggests that the pressures of restructuring encourage nurse managers to choose team members who are "'like' them more than those who are 'different'" (15). This implies that team formations in healthcare sectors in the context of restructuring frequently reproduce hierarchies of gender, "race" and ethnicity.

Some Canadian scholars have also written about the racialized impact of restructuring in healthcare (Das Gupta 1994; 1996a; Gray 1994; Lum and Williams 2000; Hagey et al. 2001). As discussed before, in the context of restructuring of healthcare in the 1990s, there was greater differentiation among nurses on the basis of length of training and passing of licensing exams, both of which became highly racialized processes. It is clear that nurses, a highly feminized workforce, became even more segmented along lines of "race," ethnicity and immigration status (Lum and Williams 2000). Nurses of colour and Black nurses were more adversely affected than white nurses by the restructuring that took place in the 1990s. Harassment frequently turned out to be a process that resulted in nurses of colour being ejected from their jobs. Some who were eligible took early retirement to escape harassment (Gray 1994), and others simply quit their job for the same reason.

In conducting this present study, a search of the ONA Law database using the keywords "race" and "racism" revealed that most race related grievances referred to arbitration were filed in the 1990s. This was confirmed by the Grievance Arbitration Tracking (GAT) system of the Association, although this database provided only general information about "discrimination" cases overall,[5] i.e., without breaking them down according to race, gender, disability or other grounds. Table 3.1 presents a breakdown of the yearly totals of "discrimination" related grievances.

One likely hypothesis accounting for this pattern is that discussed earlier: the 1990s was a decade of crisis in nursing. A number of high profile cases arose in this period that highlighted racial harassment of Black nurses within

Table 3.1 Total Discrimination Grievances, by Year

Year	Number of Grievances	Year	Number of Grievances
1980	1	1991	36
1981	0	1992	104
1982	3	1993	147
1983	14	1994	100
1984	8	1995	58
1985	8	1996	41
1986	6	1997	60
1987	9	1998	37
1988	7	1999	24
1989	17	2000	14
1990	23	2001	30

a restructuring environment. The following is a discussion of some of the more significant ones.

NURSES AT NORTHWESTERN GENERAL HOSPITAL

In 1990, seven Black nurses and one Filipino nurse employed at Northwestern General Hospital (NWGH) filed complaints with the Ontario Human Rights Commission (OHRC). They claimed that they had been subjected to racial harassment and had in some cases been fired or forced to resign as a result. The claims of the NWGH nurses were similar to the issues pointed out earlier by The Healthcare Team (Head 1985). I had the privilege of acting as a consultant for the complainants from NWGH and in that capacity was given access to materials compiled on the cases. Many of my ideas regarding how harassment works and how it is connected to systemic racism in the workplace and in society at large were developed while working on that project (Das Gupta 1994).

Apart from my analysis of harassment at NWGH, the Hospital, in conjunction with the Ontario Anti-Racism Secretariat,[6] the Ontario Ministry of Health and the Ontario Hospital Association, consulted with the Doris Marshall Institute (DMI) and Minors (1994) to produce two reports, one concerning the status of racism and another generating short- and long-term recommendations to address racism. The first report noted that nurses of colour were reluctant to provide individual or group interviews for fear of reprisals by their employer. It was reported that eleven complaints to the OHRC in 1991 were followed by seventeen further complaints, some of which were filed by staff claiming they had experienced reprisals for filing their original complaints. The Hospital denied these allegations.

On the basis of a survey that had been conducted in 1992 by a Hospital task force, DMI and Minors noted that out of 357 respondents, 26 percent reported that they had been discriminated against. Most of these were people of colour, who reported that their experience of discrimination was based on race, culture, education or country of origin.

After four years of hearings, deliberations and advocacy by members of community and labour organizations, the nurses reached a settlement, with the intervention of a provincially appointed mediator. The Hospital agreed to pay each nurse a minimum of $10,000 for mental anguish, with the biggest single payment being $100,000. Since then, other nurses of colour have come forward and filed grievances with the ONA as well as complained to the OHRC about similar experiences (Das Gupta 1996a, 1996b; Calliste 1996; Collins et al. 1997), most notably nurses at North York Branson Hospital and the Clarke Institute of Psychiatry (Depradine 1995), both of which are located in Toronto. After the landmark settlement reached by nurses at NWGH, individuals and employer institutions had to acknowledge the high costs, both personal and financial, associated with complaints of racism.

There was also a call by the Coalition for Black Nurses for a public inquiry into racism in the healthcare system and similar calls from the Christian Leadership Council, the ONA and the Canadian Labour Congress following an Anti-Racism and Healthcare Conference (Depradine 1994). Moreover, some critics want an assistant deputy minister appointed to handle anti-racism in healthcare. These demands have not been met yet.

NURSES AT BRANSON HOSPITAL

A group of non-white nurses and other healthcare staff at Branson Hospital won a settlement of $300,000 in 1995 but were prevented from speaking publicly about it due to a gag order put on them by the OHRC. They had alleged wrongful dismissal, lack of support from hospital administrators for nurses of colour and an anonymous letter sent to a Black nursing manager threatening her life (Depradine 1995a).

NURSES AT THE UNIVERSITY HEALTH NETWORK

In December 1999, Local 97 of the ONA voted to censure downtown Toronto's University Health Network (Toronto Hospital's General and Western Divisions and Princess Margaret Hospital). This vote was sanctioned by the ONA's board of directors. Local members were concerned about patient safety and care due to ongoing harassment, discrimination, poor labour relations and occupational health and safety violations. Nurses were low in morale, overworked and burned out. The Health Network had been censured several times, beginning in 1989, and again in 1991 and in 1996, the latter specifically over racism and discrimination concerns (ONA 1999). Obviously, the problems identified by nurses were not being addressed by management. Barb Wahl, ONA Provincial President, identified the problem of a poisoned environment marked by intimidation and discrimination. Equal opportunities for advancement did not exist for nurses of colour, who also frequently suffered harassment from doctors. In addition, nurses were pressured to work while they were ill under threats of being fired if they did not comply.

RESPONSES TO RACISM IN NURSING IN THE 1990S

The ONA responded to these new realities with changes in its institutional structure. In 1993, Kim Bernhardt was hired as the Research Officer in Human Rights. In the following year, the ONA's board passed a motion that up to $1 million be allocated to develop short- and long-term strategic principles necessary to address human rights and equity issues. In 1997, the Human Rights and Equity Team, comprised of ONA members, staff and management representing designated groups, was established to address human rights and equity issues affecting ONA membership. In 2001, the ONA created the Human Rights and Equity Specialist. Currently, each ONA bargaining unit has a human rights representative, and a board member carries the human rights and equity portfolio. It is noteworthy that 89 percent of the ONA members believed in 2000 that the union should work with employers to reduce discrimination in the workplace and the healthcare system (Pottins 2000).

RACISM AS "SOCIAL FORMATION" IN NURSING WORK TODAY

As critical race scholars note, there are new discourses of "race" today that-stay away from the use of "race as biology" argument prevalent in earlier years. Racism in paid workplaces is also disguised, thus making it challenging to identify, understand and combat. Despite that, racial harassment is at the basis of the grievances filed by many nurses of colour. Other forms of racism, such as attitudinal and systemic racism, are also difficult to identify since they are usually hidden behind formal workplace policies, procedures and requirements that do not appear to discriminate on their face and are not readily revealed through direct experiences. Let us refer back to Joan's case, described in the introduction.

In Joan's case, incidents that constituted harassment took the form of what one would imagine were regular manager-staff interactions. Joan's manager reminded her about her tardiness, her punctuality and her professional practice. On the face of it, these reminders from her manager seemed to be indications of Joan's incompetence as a nurse.

It was only when she was fired without due process and when she became aware of other Black nurses being treated in a similar (negative) manner compared to white nurses that Joan realized she was being racially harassed. Not only was she being verbally admonished, but a file of negative documentation was being built on her with help from co-workers. The difficulty of viewing their experiences within the larger work context and the inability to compare their experiences with that of other nurses are some of the reasons why grievors often take a long time to come to terms with their own harassment. In busy hospital settings, generally characterized by overwork, an individual does not have contact with all nurses and has no access to management files.

I argue that although there was no articulated discourse of "race" in these harassing behaviours, it is nurses of colour who are being disproportionately subjected to them. These behaviours and resulting interactions can be deconstructed to reveal a discourse steeped in notions of "race," a gendered "race" to be exact. Frequently, verbal and written responses, lack of responses and informal comments by management after the fact confirm my argument.

In my analytical report on Northwestern General Hospital (1994) and in my book *Racism and Paid Work* (1996), I describe the various ways that racial harassment of an "everyday" (Essed 1991) nature is perpetuated by managers and co-workers. My description of everyday racism in the workplace was based on my research in the garment industry, my experience with workers who had filed human rights cases and a review of literature on workplace racism. I argued that the patterns of everyday racism were all evident at NWGH. The following is a summary of these patterns:

- Targeting – a worker of colour is singled out for differential treatment, including harsher scrutiny, more severe discipline and undesirable work assignments. Joan was subjected to this.
- Scapegoating – a worker of colour or a group of them is blamed for something in the workplace and then pay the consequences for that. For instance, if there is an error made in medication of a patient, a Black nurse will be blamed for it even though there were others, including the doctor, contributing to that error.
- Excessive monitoring – a worker of colour is watched, supervised and documented. The documentation is then used against the worker as proof of incompetence. We see this in Joan's case when she was accompanied by her manager on her regular rounds and reminded of standard procedures. She was also being monitored and documented regarding her punctuality while white nurses were not being watched in a similar manner.
- Marginalization – a worker of colour is isolated or excluded from formal and informal workplace networks. This results in a sense of insecurity and exclusion from crucial information sharing at the workplace. For instance, a nurse of colour is not invited to parties given by colleagues or by her manager.
- Dispersion – workers of one ethnic or racialized group are assigned to tasks, shifts or break times away from each other in order to break their solidarity. This reduces workers' sense of security and networking capacity.
- Infantilization – a worker of colour is belittled, put down or given the message that she/he is not "good enough." In the process of being infantilized, the worker's dignity, self worth and adulthood are reduced. This often has a negative effect on the worker's ability to perform well. Joan, a senior nurse with many years of experience, was lectured on routine procedures.
- Blaming the victim – a worker of colour is often blamed for being racially harassed or abused in general. There is a denial of racism or abuse, and the immediate response of the worker to racism or abuse, such as a heated exchange of words and the resultant alienation from co-workers, are often used as a basis for discipline. There is an inability

to understand that it is human to be upset after being racially harassed. The state of being upset and resisting harassment is often interpreted as "lack of professionalism." For instance, Joan was accused of "yelling" in a similar situation.

- Bias in work allocation – differential workloads or types of work are allocated to workers of colour. In many workplaces, workers of colour are assigned the heaviest, dirtiest, most unsafe, undesirable, poorly paid, insecure jobs in relation to white workers. The resulting division of labour perpetuates marginalization described above. For instance, Black workers may be consistently assigned to night duties and to patients who need lifting due to chronic illnesses.

- Underemployment and denial of promotions – a worker of colour is denied access to training towards new job openings that are higher in status than her current job. She is refused training, upgrading or mentoring by her manager on subjective grounds while her white co-worker with less qualification and seniority is mentored and eventually promoted.

- Lack of accommodation – accommodation to disability is obstructed or denied due to a judgement made by management that the illness or disability is non-existent. Denial of accommodation may be expressed in a variety of ways, including minimizing workers' complaints or being inflexible regarding sick leave policy. The worker of colour who is denied accommodation is then found to be incompetent or set up for failure.

- Segregation – management hires workers of diverse ethnic/racial backgrounds and then channels them to work in homogenous workforces. This results in shifts, task groups and work areas being defined by ethnicity, "race" and/or gender. It is not a surprise that Joan mentions that the chronic care unit was mostly staffed by Black nurses. Management might practise differential policies for different groups of workers, thus leading to bias in work allocation and underemployment described above.

- Co-optation and selective alliances – a worker of colour or a white worker is taken on side by management and asked to spy on workers of colour or to assist in targeting or over-monitoring a worker of colour. Allying oneself with management against a co-worker may be motivated by fear of harassment, insecurity due to lay-offs or hopes of getting ahead in a competitive field. Joan was asked by her manager for information about some of her Black colleagues. When she refused to comply she became targeted herself for harassment.

- Tokenism – it is a common practice for management to deny racism by hiring one or two workers of colour in supervisory positions. Token positions are usually short-term and have limited power. Tokens might also be subjected to harassment such as underemployment, marginalization and co-optation.

Class, gender, racial and other bases of power/privilege (individually or in combination) usually characterize the perpetrator of racial harassment. It is usually an employer, manager, owner or someone in a professional role, such as a teacher, doctor or nurse. However, white co-workers and clients can also harass a professional of colour based on their racial, gender and other privileges. Similarly, an able-bodied nurse has power over a nurse with a disability. In many cases, we find a nurse of colour with a disability being harassed by white able-bodied nurses. In this case, the power and privilege that come from racialization and being differently abled intersect.

Moreover, we can see how racism operates in local work sites as "social formations" (Omi and Winant 1994). Everyday racist behaviour, which amounts to racial harassment, is allowed to continue by an institution that has entrenched systemic racism. In other words, individual perpetrators can behave in a certain manner because the procedures, policies and practices allow those behaviours to continue. In the following section, I discuss how everyday racism is linked with systemic racism in the hiring, promotion, training, performance appraisal, disciplining and firing policies, procedures and practices of hospitals and how these practices in turn are related to racist discourse. I argue that everyday behaviours towards Black female nurses can be deconstructed to reveal both systemic racism and racist-sexist discourses about women of colour and Black women.

Everyday racist behaviours experienced by Black nurses occur within a backdrop of anti-Black racism and sexism, specifically racist discourses about Black women workers that emanated during the slavery of African peoples. Discourses refer to bodies of ideas that are characterized by apparent coherence and theoretical consistency and that have been given authoritative status through academic, professional, government or other accepted approval processes. Usually, discourses reproduce the status quo. For instance, such discourses as equal opportunity, freedom of speech and meritocracy have been utilized to maintain the way things are, including racism, sexism and other social injustices.

Segregation, e.g., the over-representation of Black workers in hospital chronic care units, considered heavy and undesirable work, and under-representation in the intensive care units and operating rooms, seen as more desirable, is to be understood in the context of biased recruitment and streaming methods. These are accomplished through word-of-mouth hiring, inconsistent outreach methods and interviews conducted by individuals, almost always white, lacking in cross-cultural and anti-racist training, with inconsistent patterns of reference requirements. The resultant segregation of workers and bias in work allocation in the hospital reflects and in turn reproduces anti-Black racial discourse in which Black women are seen to be suited to physically demanding, yet mentally less challenging, work and are expected to be happy with this arrangement.

Another form of segregation, e.g., the overwhelming whiteness of management in hospitals, is produced by biased promotional, mentoring and leadership training opportunities, as well as by racially biased performance appraisal systems, which disqualify nurses from promotions. For instance, vague and subjective criteria are often used to evaluate the performance level of nurses. Examples cited in some of my studies (1996, 1994) are "communication skills," "interpersonal skills" and "leadership." These criteria are not described in any detail so that the manager appraising a nurse is left to interpret these descriptors in her/his own way. This leaves room for subjectivity and thus bias. How would a white manager untrained in cross-cultural issues judge a nurse of colour who speaks English with a non-dominant accent or dialect? How would the same manager judge a nurse of colour who is not cordial with some of her colleagues because she has received rude or racist treatment from them? Would a manager view a nurse's assertiveness in standing up to sexism or racism as insubordination or leadership?

The methods used to fill leadership positions are frequently inconsistent, ad hoc and based on the subjective orientation of one person, usually white. It is not uncommon to find that a junior white nurse will be mentored and trained for promotion while a senior Black nurse will be passed over.

The nurses of the Healthcare Team (Head 1985), for instance, alleged that they were allocated to more menial jobs, streamed into less preferred units and under-represented in supervisory and management positions. Promotions were often not accessible to them as they were more likely to be subjected to biased performance evaluations. The latter often led to disciplinary hearings and to dismissals rather than to follow-ups and improvements. It is noteworthy that the College of Nurses (CNO), the provincial regulatory body for nurses, was described as not having representation either from non-white members or even white members from the lower levels of the nursing hierarchy. It was predominantly made up of white women who had previously held administrative and executive positions in hospitals. Many of these problems continue, with Gustafson (2002) noting that the CNO was the "domain of white women," particularly in its executive levels.

An overwhelming white management, untrained in anti-racism and cross-cultural approaches, is the context for a variety of racially biased stereotypes and prejudices consciously or unconsciously operating about nurses of colour. These attitudes influence interactions between management and staff and among staff nurses. For instance, workers of colour are often perceived as "out of control," "irrational" and "threatening." These are based in historical perceptions of non-white peoples as less than human, wild and animal-like, uncivilized and therefore to be feared and kept in check. Experiences of targeting, dispersing, marginalization, co-optation and selective alliances emanate from such fears.

These fears are particularly heightened when workers of colour seek to enforce their rights as workers or as racialized peoples by confrontation, speaking out or filing grievances. Through such demands workers of colour threaten the existing power structures including the behaviours and attitudes of managers as well as their employing institutions. In such situations, management retaliates by targeting, disciplining and, if all else fails, by firing them. In most of these cases, the employing institution backs management. It is not a coincidence that many nurses of colour who have confronted a co-worker, patient or manager or who have filed grievances alleging racism have faced negative performance appraisals or been suspended or fired (DMI and Minors 1994; Hagey, Choudhry et al. 2001).

Disciplinary procedures and practices can also be examples of how systemic racism works. As discussed before, white workers and workers of colour are disciplined differently. Workers of colour committing minor errors are often disciplined while white workers are not. White workers committing errors are often given support and education to improve while workers of colour are simply monitored more often, set up for failure and documented. These differentials happen largely due to the subjectivity and vagueness that imbue the disciplinary process. Again, as in the case of recruitment, hiring and performance appraisal systems, discipline is also imposed by a manager who is usually white.

Historical stereotypes about people of colour include their alleged inherent dishonesty. This stereotype gives rise to management susceptibility to scapegoating and to denying racism and disability claims. The worker of colour's culpability is often assumed in situations where a problem or irregularity has occurred in the workplace. Such accusations can be used to deny them privileges or opportunities given to white workers or even to discipline them.

Asking for the acknowledgement of racism or disability by workers of colour is often seen to be a result of "excitability" and "over-sensitivity" at best and "dishonesty", "laziness" and "incompetence" at worst. Their complaints are often viewed as exaggerated and thus untrue. With such practices, racism and disability are denied. Depending on the persistence of workers of colour and thus the seriousness of their challenge to authority, they may be further subjected to targeting and marginalizing practices.

The general tendency to deny racism is systemically supported by the absence or ineffective implementation of an anti-harassment policy and accompanying procedures in employing institutions. If there is no policy in place to handle a complaint of racial harassment, it is usually met with denial or dealt with inadequately by management. If there is a policy in place, management may not be trained or guided to use it effectively. Management's general reluctance to entertain the veracity of a complaint is further conditioned by the ineptitude of the procedure to handle such complaints.

LIMITATION OF INSTITUTIONAL RESPONSES TO RACISM

In response to human rights cases which it dealt with, and through consultations with community advocates, organizations and experts, the OHRC has developed impressive conceptualizations of modern-day racism in Canada. However, application and implementation of new insights have been less than adequate. For instance, the Ontario *Human Rights Code* (2001) contemplates that an employer, whether it is a corporation, union or occupational association, may be liable for racial harassment perpetrated by an employee or employees, particularly management employees. This is referred to as "corporate responsibility." In theory, this could be used effectively to counteract systemic racism perpetuated by employers. Unfortunately, the proactive rhetoric of the Code does not necessarily translate to the advantage of a person subjected to racial harassment, even when the harassment is overt. The case of Emilda Shaffer,[7] a Black nurse in Ottawa, who was racially slurred and subsequently slapped by a white co-worker in 1981, is a case in point. The Humans Right Tribunal ruled that the employer had no liability since the nurse was racially harassed and assaulted by a co-worker rather than a supervisor and that the "anemic" response by the employer was appropriate given the nature of the incident, which was judged to be less serious than if she had been assaulted by a supervisor.

Calliste (1996) notes that both the ONA and the OHRC were initially reluctant to deal with the complaints of racial harassment from nurses at NWGH as systemic and that this reluctance led to the formation of the Coalition for Black Nurses, initiated by the Congress of Black Women of Canada and Nurses and Friends Against Discrimination (NAFAD). Following the advocacy efforts of these groups, the complaints of the eight nurses were investigated by the OHRC as a systemic racism complaint, the first and only time this has been done.

Human rights commissions have been guilty of passive racism, that is, by their inaction in the face of racial harassment. In addition to the OHRC's initial non-supportive response to the nurses from NWGH, Calliste (1996) highlights two cases, one in Ontario and another in Quebec, where provincial commissions failed in their mandate to address human rights violations. In the first case, an official with the OHRC, who was assigned to investigate a complaint by a Black nurse, decided to assist the defendant hospital to build its case because of personal friendships with some of its personnel. The nurse's case was dismissed (Maylor 1987). Although irregularities in procedure were noted by the Ombudsman's Office, there was no further action taken by the OHRC.

In the second case, a mediator-investigator from the Quebec Human Rights Commission (QHRC) demonstrated bias by holding a number of meetings with the defendant hospital's lawyer and personnel director in the absence of the lawyer of the Quebec Association of Black Nurses, one of whose members was the complainant.

In 1994, the NAFAD held a protest in Toronto against the OHRC's invoking of Section 34 of the *Human Rights Code*, which allows the commission to dismiss complaints if they can be dealt with in another jurisdiction (Fanfair 1994). The NAFAD alleged that a significant number of racial harassment complaints were being thrown out by the OHRC in this manner. In addition, they pointed out other systemic problems with the OHRC, including long delays in processing complaints, lack of public accountability and inadequate funding.

Three years later, the ONA and Parkdale Community Legal Services Inc. held a news conference where they charged the OHRC again for using Section 34 to refuse action on complaints made by unionized female workers (Donkoh 1997). At this time four women, including three nurses, were taking the OHRC to court for judicial review of their decisions to dismiss various complaints. The three women had been subjected to harassment on the basis of race, sex and disability. The applications for judicial review were subsequently dismissed.

RESEARCH METHODS

Having discussed the theoretical and historical literature around anti-Black racism in nursing in Canada, we are now in a position to delve into researching current issues and experiences in this area. However, before we embark on that, this section provides a discussion of my research methods.

As discussed in the introductory chapter, I was approached by the Ontario Nurses' Association (ONA) in 2001 to research and write a document on systemic racism in this profession. Thus, from the inception of this project, there has been close consultation with ONA staff concerning research design and methods. Given the complex and layered nature of racism in healthcare settings, I had to resort to a variety of research techniques, chiefly of a qualitative nature. In addition, in order to reveal the continuum between everyday racist behaviours of white nurses, administrators and other healthcare workers, systemic racism and common-sensical attitudes of prejudice and stereotyping, an indepth case study of one nurse of colour seemed necessary. I selected an illustrative case of a nurse who had gone to arbitration. In doing this, I was restricted in terms of what information I could reveal as I was operating under ethical protocols. For instance, I was informed by the ONA that I could only refer to information presented in the final arbitration reports rather than other case particulars that exist in the file. Apart from the case study selected for detailed examination, I examined documents related to other incidents of alleged racial harassment by ONA members. This documentary research resulted in content and discourse analysis of arbitration proceedings.

Towards the beginning of the research, I consulted with Darla Rhyme, of the Institute of Social Research (ISR) at York University (Toronto), who is an expert on qualitative research design. She suggested using a short survey tool to acquire an overall picture of the problem I was studying. This would capture issues I may not have thought of initially. She also suggested names of colleagues[8] who had conducted similar surveys on the topic of sexual harassment, and their survey instruments were made available to me.

Although an enormous amount of information was gathered through these methods, they were limited in that the voices of the nurses were muted. Smith (1992: 17) called for a political economy that "explore[s] and display[s] the properties and movement of the complex of powers, forces and relations that are at work in our everyday/everynight worlds."[9] Experience becomes a concrete everyday/everynight expression of political economy, one that is inclusive of those who are at the margins of the formal economy. It is this concept of the everyday worlds of women workers of colour that I wished to explore in this study in conjunction with how formal texts such as arbitration reports spoke about them.

In line with Smith's (1992) critique of the documentary construction of reality, I realized that documents, particularly legal arbitration and grievance settlement reports, had a way of sifting out or truncating subjective experience, or classifying it as invalid. Moreover, given the lack of understanding of systemic racism among arbitration board members, apart from a minority of dissenting members, the arbitration reports overall had no analysis of that aspect of racism. Thus, the documents to which I had access, although invaluable, did not yield information that was central to my study, that is, the nature of everyday racism, which operates subtly. Nor did they provide much information on how systemic racism operates. Because of limitations of both the documents and the survey I also conducted indepth interviews with nurses who experienced racial harassment, including some who filed grievances.

Of all the forms of racism, the most difficult to study is systemic racism as it requires a thorough systems review of an institution. I had neither the time nor resources to this. Although the arbitration files contained some such information, I could only reveal information contained in the arbitration reports, which were public documents. The survey did yield patterns of discrimination that nurses of colour experience in their working lives compared to white nurses, which is a result of systemic racism within employment. This information was further confirmed through indepth interviews. Anticipating that sceptics would question the subjective nature of interview materials as well as of survey responses, I fell back on my (1994) systemic study of the Northwestern General Hospital (NWGH), which had been based on formal documents generated by the hospital itself.

The following is a descriptive listing of all the research methods that I used for the study.

Documentary Analysis

A search was conducted of ONA Law (referred to before) using keywords such as "discrimination," "racism" and "race." This generated sixteen arbitration decisions and three grievance settlements, all except one being from the 1990s. In some cases, multiple grievances had been submitted by one nurse. The key word searches did not capture cases that had been resolved before being referred to arbitration. The concentration of grievances in the 1990s can be attributed to the nursing crisis in the late 1980s and 1990s. Other reasons were also offered by the ONA, including increased member and public education on the topic.

Documents in the nineteen grievance files, including arbitration decisions, case particulars and "expert" reports, were reviewed and analyzed. Each arbitration report was reviewed, and information was noted under the following categories: types of alleged harassment, systemic issues, grievor's response, management response, effects of harassment on grievor and final outcome.

Survey

A short survey instrument was designed to capture a snapshot of workplace experiences of nurses of colour who are members of the ONA. The survey instrument as well as a consent form to be used for future interviews were reviewed and approved by York University's Human Participants Review Sub-Committee.

The survey instrument was piloted at an information meeting of nurses in the community and subsequently distributed at the Racially Diverse Caucus at the Provincial Coordinators' Meeting of the ONA in November 2001 in Toronto. Approximately thirty surveys were distributed with a brief explanation of their purpose. Respondents were asked to mail or fax it back to me or to hand it in at the end of the meeting. The response rate was disappointing as only eight were received.

Other ways of distributing the survey instrument were explored. Karen Sandercock, ONA Human Rights and Equity Specialist, informed me about a series of meetings with nurses that were being organized as part of another research project, "Integrating Accountability for Employment Equity in Canada," funded by the Race Relations Foundation. The principal investigator[10] of that project agreed to allow me to distribute the survey at these community meetings. This proved to be much more successful. Sixty-two

Table 3.2 Respondents to the Survey by Ethnicity/Race

Ethnicity/Race*	Numbers	Percent
Black/African	62	10.5
Asian	60	10.1
South Asian	18	3
Aboriginal/First Nations	1	0.2
Central/South American	7	1.2
White/European	311	52.4
Other**	122	20.6
Not Identified	12	2
Total	593	100

* Respondents were asked to self-identify
** Many of these are mixed raced women. The large percentage of nurses who marked "other" needs to be investigated further for future research.

Table 3.3 Respondents to the Survey by Gender

Gender	Numbers	Percent
Female	571	96.3
Male	17	2.9
No Answer	5	0.8
Total	593	100

surveys were filled out at these meetings, most of them by nurses of colour.

One error occurred initially in the surveys distributed through the latter workshops: I did not ask the nurses to identify their designation or their current job title. As a result, there was no way to ascertain whether they were RNs, RPNs, non-union and managerial staff or UCPs. Subsequently, this omission was corrected. Also, midway through the surveying process, I added a few additional questions concerning educational level because I felt that they might generate useful information.

Although the surveys generated rich information about the experiences of nurses of colour, I felt that it would be valuable to hear also from white nurses as a comparative group. To facilitate this, Karen Sandercock arranged for the survey to be mailed to all of the ONA's membership. Accordingly, about 40,000 members received a copy of the survey, and they were given two weeks in which to return the completed survey. On Ms. Sandercock's advice, a few additional questions, particularly for white nurses, were added.

Utilizing all these outreach methods, I received 593 responses overall.

One of the reasons for this low response is that nurses had to mail back the surveys on their own volition, supplying their own envelope and stamp, although faxing was also an option. The latter method would not result in a cost to the member; however, it could be perceived as not providing them with full confidentiality. A number of members expressed annoyance at having to pay for the mailing of the surveys in their written comments or by phone. Despite the low survey response relative to the total membership, there was more than enough information generated to fulfil my objective of obtaining comparative data about racism from white nurses. It must be remembered though that the sample is not representative of the nursing population as a whole. It was self-selected, not random.[11] Therefore, the information generated cannot be used to generalize about the entire nursing population. Nonetheless, the survey was successful in acquiring responses from a diverse group of nurses from all over the province, and it does confirm that racism is a serious concern among nurses, particularly those of colour.

The ISR, which provides statistical services, coded the results on an SPSS Program and provided frequency tables with cross-tabulations for further analysis. These are discussed in Chapter 5. Tables 3.2 and 3.3 provide demographic breakdowns of those who responded to the survey.

Interviews

Those surveyed both through the ONA and through the community meetings were asked whether they would be willing to be interviewed. For those nurses contacted through community meetings, a short form was designed for them to indicate in writing whether they would be interested in being interviewed. A number of nurses of colour indicated such a willingness to be contacted for this purpose and left their phone number, e-mail or other contact information. Fourteen nurses were interviewed in person or over the phone. The interviews were taped and transcribed. Names and identifying information were changed to maintain confidentiality and anonymity.

Statistics

Inquiries were made to see if demographic data could be acquired from the National Institute of Health Information (NIHI), which is designated to maintain a statistical database on nursing. I was advised that they do not collect statistics on race or ethnicity. The NIHI referred us to Statistics Canada for such information. This method was not fruitful either. The College of Nurses in Toronto was also contacted for statistical information, and they informed me that a special request would have to be made to generate this kind of data.

Library Searches

Extensive library research was conducted to identify historical and secondary literature on racism in nursing both in Canada and outside Canada.

Through these five methods, i.e., documentary analysis, surveys, interviews, limited statistical data and review of secondary literature, a fairly comprehensive overview was developed concerning racism in nursing. The next three chapters present and analyze the findings resulting from the application of all these methods.

NOTES

1. A follow-up study (Murray and Frisina 1988) noted a high rate of resignations all over Canada.
2. Interview with Colleen Ionson, Labour Relations Officer in ONA, Hamilton, May 6, 2002.
3. The proxy comparison method refers to pay equity measures undertaken by the comparison of a predominantly or wholly female workplace to a similar large workplace nearby where pay inequities between men and women have already been identified. The proxy method was legislated through Bill 102 passed in 1993 by the NDP government in Ontario.
4. A Charter challenge was filed in 2001 by CUPE, ONA, OPSEU, SEIU, USWA and four women.
5. These numbers are only an indication of the numbers of grievances handled by the ONA during these years. They were generated by a search of GAT using such keywords as "discrimination," "discharge" and "unreasonable policy." GAT does not indicate the grounds of discrimination generally, although a manual review reveals that "disability" is often noted. Even though "race" was added to the list of keywords in approximately 1996, it is apparent that it was not used consistently in identifying the files. The reasons behind this omission are worth exploration as they may indicate the ways in which arbitration boards often interpret race-related grievances as arising due to labour-management conflict or personal conflict rather than due to racism.
6. This government body established under the NDP government of the time was dismantled by the PC government that subsequently came to power.
7. See *Shaffer v. Treasury Board of Canada* 1984.
8. These included Linda Briskin and Nancy Mandell.
9. Dorothy Smith's work has been inspirational to many feminist academics, for example, the authors in Campbell and Manicom (1995).
10. Dr. Rebecca Hagey, School of Nursing, University of Toronto.
11. A random sample would require information on the racial/ethnic breakdown of the nursing population in Ontario, which does not exist currently.

4.   ONE NURSE'S STORY

This chapter is about racism and, in particular, what it looks like today in the context of racial harassment in paid work. How are racial discourses reproduced in the age of equity, human rights, anti-racism and diversity? As argued before, systemic racism is frequently not revealed through personal experiences or observations and requires theorizing to develop a conceptual understanding of what racism is and how it works. This does not mean that overt racism in the workplace is a thing of the past. It still manifests itself and affects the same bodies, but it is rationalized using different discourses compared to those prevalent in past times, which were generally based on biological and cultural arguments of inferiority. In order to concretize my ideas, I present the story of Evelyn, a Black nurse working with East York Health Unit who filed several grievances through the ONA during the 1990s.[1]

> Evelyn first suspected that something was not quite right during a performance appraisal four years before she took early retirement to put an end to her harassment. In that appraisal, she was marked "satisfactory." However, her manager criticized her over her communication skills. This was the context within which subsequent incidents, conversations and interactions took place between Evelyn and her manager and co-workers.
>
> A few months later, she was suspended for two weeks without pay and moved to a different community setting as a disciplinary measure for allegedly not acting appropriately in her role as a nurse. She lost her grievance over her suspension.
>
> Approximately two years later she was given an "unsatisfactory" performance appraisal as well as a thirty-day improvement contract. The negative performance reviews continued a month later. She filed grievances for her negative performance appraisals to be removed from her files and be destroyed and asked that the employer stop requiring extra supervision, work and remedial action that was not required of other nurses. She alleged that her negative performance appraisals as well as the so-called improvement contract constituted racial harassment. She was given further suspensions for failing to fulfil requirements in the improvement contract. The employer decided to extend the improvement contract further.
>
> She filed further grievances to have more recent negative appraisals removed from her files and destroyed and to be reimbursed for monies, seniority and service lost due to the suspensions. She also asked for an end to the over-supervision, harassment and discrimination.

Two months later, she resigned. In her resignation letter, she stated that she was resigning because of the discriminatory behaviour directed towards her. Once she resigned, Evelyn was no longer subjected to performance reviews.

Approximately two years later, when the Arbitration Board met to decide on all the grievances described above, Evelyn's employers informed the ONA that they would remove the documents as desired from Evelyn's file and that she would be compensated for lost wages and benefits for the periods of suspensions. In addition, they would implement recommendations concerning human rights awareness and conflict resolution in the workplace.

The ONA sought for Evelyn to be reinstated in her employment as further relief from her grievances. The ONA argued that the continuing discrimination and harassment created a poisoned environment for Evelyn, affecting her health and ultimately forcing her to resign. Unfortunately, the latter argument was not persuasive of board members, who decided that the resignation was not related to her other grievances over her performance appraisals. They further stated that Evelyn could have filed another grievance and argued that her resignation was not a result of discriminatory conduct and that it amounted to constructive dismissal. It is noteworthy that there was a partial dissent from one of the members, who stated that the reasoning used by the board was "far too narrow and unduly technical." She further stated that the grievances were not only about Evelyn's performance reviews, but rather about discriminatory treatment, arguing that the latter should have been the focus of the reasoning behind the board's final decision.[2] Evelyn's story and my analysis in the following paragraphs are presented as a counter-narrative to the one that was submitted by the majority of the arbitration board members. The narrative of the one dissenting board member also substantiates the counter-narrative. Delgado and Stefancic (2000: 60) and other critical race theorists write that the legal arena is a terrain of struggle between stories of ingroups (those in dominance) and outgroups (the marginalized). The stories or narratives of dominant groups create a sense of community among themselves and maintain an understanding of their own dominance as natural. "The stories of outgroups aim to subvert that reality" (60). Counter-narratives can "shatter complacency and challenge the status quo" (61).

Readers might ask why they should believe Evelyn's counter-narrative rather than the official narrative, where she was judged to be an incompetent nurse and whose treatment by her employers was judged not to have been marked by racial discrimination. I would respond by saying that Evelyn's experience is not unique. Hers is a dramatic example of racial harassment in Ontario; however, the patterns of harassment she experienced are fairly common. Her story is corroborated by hundreds of other stories of Black nurses and nurses of colour, a few of whom won their grievances, but the majority of whom did not.

Evelyn was subjected to a number of everyday behaviours by her management that included marginalization and infantilization, biased work allocation, blame for her own victimization and excessive monitoring and documentation. These behaviours are examples of everyday racism (see previous chapter), and they cumulatively had an adverse impact upon Evelyn's professional and personal life.

Evelyn was subjected to targeting, which happens when one worker is singled out for differential treatment, including harsher scrutiny, more severe discipline and undesirable work assignments. This often happens to nurses of colour who are confident, capable and outspoken.

The first suspension that Evelyn experienced appears to have been a result of scapegoating, another example of racist managerial action. She was disciplined for not providing first aid to a child who sustained an eye injury and who eventually lost vision in that eye permanently. When Evelyn had been asked to provide first aid, she had insisted that the child needed to be taken to the hospital to be seen by a doctor. For a variety of reasons, this action was not taken immediately by other adults present on the scene, which included a vice principal and two secretaries of the school where the injury took place. But, Evelyn was apparently the only one vilified and subjected to discipline.

In addition, I believe that Evelyn was subjected to infantilization, which as discussed before occurs when a worker of colour is belittled, put down or given the message that she/he is not "good enough." In the process of being infantilized, the worker's dignity, self worth and adulthood are reduced. This often has a negative effect on their ability to perform well. In early racist discourse based on biological or genetic reasoning (Banton 1987), Black people were assumed to be undeveloped compared to Europeans, more childlike and therefore in need of guidance and teaching. Moreover, they were assumed to be intellectually inferior and hence good only for physical work. These notions are reproduced with infantilization and excessive monitoring. Evelyn was excessively monitored, particularly following the unsatisfactory performance appraisal and the subsequent improvement contract. Her grievances sought to remove negative documentation from her file. As discussed before, typically, the documentation resulting from excessive monitoring of nurses of colour is later used against them as proof of incompetence. It is understandable how excessive monitoring itself can cause a worker to become anxious and make more mistakes than usual.

With all these requirements, Evelyn was being set up to fail. This kind of harassment can wear out a person and negatively affect her confidence, which in turn would hinder her ability to perform well. I can see how any person would be found incompetent at the end of such a horrendous process. In Evelyn's case, she decided to resign and take early retirement in order to escape this situation.

As discussed in the last chapter, many writers have illustrated the fact that the racism of today does not include a discourse of "race" or of biological inferiority (Henry 2000; Jakubowski 1997; Kirkham 1998). They have referred to this racism as "new" racism, "democratic" racism or racism of the new right. A discourse of "nationhood," "fiscal crisis" or "merit" has replaced the early language of biological race. People are otherized not because they are deemed to be biologically different, but because they are outsiders to the nation, because the state cannot afford them or because they are not meritorious. Refugees, undocumented workers and even landed immigrants are considered to be outsiders, and treating them differently and unfairly is justified in the name of nationalism, national security, equal opportunity and the economy, just as biological inferiority justified enslavement or genocide in the past. As discussed in Chapter 2, categories such as "immigrant" and "refugee" are highly racialized in common-sensical terms, becoming code words for referring to people of colour rather than to white outsiders. Jakubowski (1997) calls this "de-racialization," a discursive practice that does not use explicitly racist categories but which has racist effects.

Similarly, today's racism from employers involves a discourse of individual incompetence or individual pathology. A worker of colour is subjected to everyday racism, then found to be incompetent and, finally, terminated or forced to resign, as in Evelyn's case. Or, a worker of colour is pathologized as having "an anger problem" or being "psychologically unstable." However, when deconstructed, everyday managerial practices apparently based on objective notions of merit and competency reveal stereotypes about non-whites from the days of slavery and colonialism. In other words, there are layers of discourses (old and new) operating here, complementing one another. Delgado and Stefancic (2000) call this "business-as-usual forms of racism that people of colour confront everyday and that accounts for much misery, alienation and despair" (xvi).

The problem is that arbitration board members are by and large not trained to conduct such deconstructive exercises; nor do they examine individual grievances as indicative of systemic problems. In relation to her first grievance, Evelyn had reported that her colleagues in the school setting were not friendly towards her and that she had become immobilized when the child, who was black, came in with an eye injury due to racial anxiety. She also reported that the school was 80 percent non-white, while the staff and administration were all white. The board decision states that Evelyn's reaction was "incomprehensible" and that "her number one priority was to comfort herself and not look after the child." It further stated that there was no evidence that Evelyn or the child were victims of racism. Evelyn was vilified as a heartless and selfish woman, only concerned about herself, without any maternal or protective instincts with regard to the child. These are tropes about Black women, which when invoked nullify them as females based on the standards of white femininity. This nullification has particular relevance for nursing as that occupation is highly gendered, with women historically cast into that role due to their alleged selfless care-giving and nurturing traits.

Without an approach that considers systemic racism, one cannot reveal the fact that management practices such as pathologization or infantilization are practised mainly against workers of colour and that there is an adverse impact on them as a result. Evelyn's grievances were dealt with as performance problems rather than as systemic racism problems. This reasoning also led to the finding that her resignation was not connected to her grievances around performance appraisals. The refusal or inability to name racism on the part of the majority of board members illustrates once again one of the foundational principles of critical race theorists, that is, "racism is normal, not aberrant.... Because racism is an ingrained feature of our landscape, it looks ordinary and natural to persons in the culture" (Delgado and Stefancic 2000: xvi). I might add that it appears particularly ordinary and natural[3] to those in racially privileged positions.

Everyday behaviours towards workers of colour can be linked to systemic racism. Evelyn's management, which suspended her as a result of the "eye injury" incident, was overwhelmingly white, a result of biased promotional, mentoring, leadership training opportunities and racially biased performance appraisal systems that disqualified nurses like her from promotions. As noted, vague and subjective criteria (communication skills, interpersonal skills) are often used to evaluate the performance level of nurses. In Evelyn's case, her communication skills were repeatedly pointed out as being deficient and contributing to her incompetence as a nurse.

Lest anyone should think that Evelyn's story is exaggerated, the next chapter presents stories from hundreds of other nurses whose narratives provide a chorus of voices that speak to the reality of racism in nursing. Evelyn's story should be read within that larger context.

NOTES

1. This story and the subsequent discussion were presented by me in a paper titled "Understanding Racial Discrimination," at the Second Annual Human Rights Symposium: Focus on Racial Discrimination, May 22 and 23, 2003, Osgoode Hall Law School of York University, Toronto.
2. *Re: East York Health Unit v. Ontario Nurses' Association* 56 LAC (4th) 1996.
3. "Ordinary" and "natural" refer to things that are seen to be "unproblematic."

5. NURSES SPEAK OUT

The survey conducted for this research was very effective in providing an overview of how racism impacts nurses of colour and poignantly reveals the different experiences of nurses of colour and of white nurses as well as differences among various groups of nurses of colour based on ethnic origin. This chapter tabulates and analyzes the responses of nurses to my survey questions and provides excerpts from the indepth interviews conducted with nurses of colour as well as from documentary research conducted at the ONA. The information presented here is both qualitative and quantitative.

EVERYDAY RACISM

In the survey conducted for this study, nurses were asked if they had ever been made to feel uncomfortable because of their race, colour or ethnicity. A startling 41 percent (245 out of 593) replied in the affirmative. When cross-tabulated by racial identity, it became clear that most nurses of colour had answered yes to this question. Eighty-two percent of Black/African Canadian nurses, 80 percent of Asian Canadian nurses, 50 percent of South Asian Canadian nurses and 57 percent of Central/South American Canadian nurses said that they had been made to feel uncomfortable due to race, colour or ethnicity. Even 25 percent of white/European Canadian nurses answered "yes," and although this is much lower than the percentages for non-white nurses, it is a significant proportion. Clearly, racialization or "race thinking" in the workplace is a major reality for non-white nurses and for many white nurses in Ontario.

LANGUAGE AND ACCENT

Many nurses elaborated on the reason for their discomfort. It was interesting that several of these elaborations dealt with language and accent. Asha, a South Asian nurse, reported being made fun of because of her pronunciation and a related incident becoming an ongoing joke among her colleagues and the nurse in charge. The following are comments from other nurses:

> I was told (in a letter) that my English is unclear. (Asian nurse)

> I come from English speaking country and I have spoken English all my life but because I'm black, they think you know nothing… They sometimes make fun of me when I am talking on the phone…
>
> It is so unfortunate that white people look down on you so much. Even though they talk about cultural sensitivity, they do not apply them. I strongly suggest cultural sensitivity issues during orientation. Sometimes even at report, they do not *even attempt* to pronounce a patient's name just

> because it is a foreign name even while you are there at report. One day a nurse told me because I have braided hair that was why I did not hear her. We certainly have a long way to go. (Black/African nurse)

These two testimonies illustrate that racialization most often involves the body or the physical attributes of a person. In these cases, it involved interpreting the nurses' manner of speaking English (i.e., their voices), their names or their "braided hair" as differentiating elements and as points of ridicule or negative assessment. In addition, this nurse points out "new" or "democratic" racism, where one finds the co-existence of "cultural sensitivity" programs at an institutional level and everyday racism, which demonstrates a total lack of cultural sensitivity on the part of the nurse making the comments. In this case, it is not clear whether the culturally insensitive remark was made by a white nurse or not. However, the comments can be attributed to a nurse who is not Black. There is nothing exclusive about racist discourses in that anyone, be they white or non-white, can internalize and articulate them. However, most of the time, when such insensitive comments are made, the person committing them is in a position of power in order to have a comfort or safety level within which to articulate them.

Another Black nurse reported that there was an unusually high level of curiosity about her boyfriend's racial and ethnic background:

> What they were trying to do, was that they were trying to size me up because I was born and raised in Canada and I'm a middle… my family is middle class, they just wanted to know what kind of men that I would be seeking out to date. So, basically they're looking to also put me in a category. Would I date a Black guy, a white guy… like what kinda guy do I date?

Trying to "put her in a category" was a result of the fact that Colleen does not fit the stereotypical Black woman in the white psyche. This created anxiety and curiosity among her colleagues. She was born in Canada, was middle class and spoke fluent English with a "Canadian" accent. Was she a part of the "in" group or outside it? Moreover, the sexuality of people of colour has historically been an object of curiosity for "race" theorists (Solomos and Back 1996). The fear of miscegenation and/or desire for the "other" have been contradictory aspects characterizing contact between whites and non-whites in colonial, post-colonial and slavery-based economies. The desire to categorize an ambiguously marked Black nurse rises out of racializing practices that people engage in, which involve viewing the world and people in it through the "race" lens. This exemplifies how race ideology, specifically racial categorization, is a way in which people make sense of and gain a sense of control and predictability in their lives. What is interesting is that everyday, commonplace interactions even today between whites and Blacks become saturated with centuries old, historically derived discourses.

Other nurses reported not being recognized for their skills, expertise, language fluency and nursing knowledge and a general dismissive or non-preferred attitude on the part of patients and managers. Nurses of colour were often made to feel worthless. I would describe these as infantilizing experiences. For example, Harriet, a Chinese Canadian nurse, said that she was often referred to as a "little Chinese nurse" or as "a little girl… not as a professional person." She adds that this image of her not only reflected racialization, but also her gender and age status. Some patients[1] clearly stated their preference for a white nurse, even if the white nurse was junior and that preference was catered to by management. Consider the following testimony from Colleen, who was presented in the introductory chapter:

> A couple of times, family would ask if I am the real nurse and I told them… RN means Real Nurse, something like that or I would say, they would think that I am… sort of like the health care aide or assistant. They wouldn't think that I was the person in charge. When I had a supervisory job, I think I shocked a few people because I think they wanted to complain about a nurse of colour… and then they… find out the nursing supervisor's of colour… somehow they became quiet. They never lodged a complaint.

In a similar vein, Amanda, also a Black nurse, says:

> Patients and their families would actually expressly tell me, oh, I would like to see the nurse in charge and when I said I'm the nurse in charge, it was evident that they did not expect that it would be me. Or, I've had patients tell me not to touch them with my Black hands or, if a patient rings and I go in, there would be some snarky joke about where are you from… where they would not have approached a Caucasian nurse like that.

Blackness in a person is associated in common-sensical racist terms with roles that are servile, "lower than" and inferior compared to whiteness. Thus, a Black nurse in charge is confusing for a person who is steeped in racial ways of thinking. Moreover, her Blackness also marks her as "dirty," "polluted" and thus unfit or dangerous to touch. This takes on a heightened significance in a setting where patients are there to fight germs and become healthy. To make matters more complicated, racial thinking is not only a monopoly of white people. As mentioned before, non-white and white are equally affected by the same discourses. Whether we internalize them or critique them usually depends on who we are, how we are affected by these discourses and whether we feel safe to enunciate them or act on those grounds.

A non-white person such as Amanda being asked "where are you from" reveals discourses of nationhood where whiteness is associated with Canadian-ness and non-whiteness with being an immigrant or refugee, who by extrapolation is a non-Canadian and an "outsider." Dua (1999: 7) notes that this logic hides the complex history of how Canada became a "white settler society" where one's ability to "become Canadian" was tied to one's "race" or skin colour.

Amanda continues to talk about an experience with a doctor:

> I think he was treating the role of [nurses] like a maid… thinking that I should pick up after him and do for him and I explained that [it] was not my role and he had a big thing about that… I noticed that he never had a problem with the other nurses… to the point where he actually went and reported me to the… to the supervisor… who came up to the floor and said, Amanda, I apologize for him… this is not our expectations.

Verbal and non-verbal behaviours often accompany these patterns, such as not being addressed, being talked down to, or being sworn at or shouted at. Brand (1999: 90) writes:

> "Black women's work" today looks like this: cleaning white people's houses, bathrooms and hotel rooms; serving white people's breakfast, lunch and dinner in private homes, in office cafeterias, hospitals; lifting, feeding minding, sweeping, boxing, scouring, washing, cooking.

She further adds that "institutionalized domestic work" characterizes Black women's work. The doctor who expected Amanda to be "a maid" was operating with such racist-sexist-classist conceptions of what Black women ought to do in hospitals. Again his racial status is not clear, but as discussed before his power base as a doctor gives him the latitude to express such ideas, whether he is white or non-white. Amanda's experience of being treated like a maid and Brand's observations about Black women's work address the question I raised in the introductory chapter about how the labour of nurses of colour may be viewed within heterosexual familial relations that seem to exist between (white) doctors and (white) nurses. Within this "family" discourse, nurses of colour (Black women, in this case) may be seen as maids and servants.

Although in the incident described by Amanda, her supervisor backed her up, they often do not. In another incident a patient's family member complained that the "Black nurse" did not feed her mother. Amanda's supervisor backed up the patient's relative in that case despite Amanda's assertion that the patient could feed herself and doing so would help with her rehabilitation. The patient's relative asserted "you are there to serve my mother," and Amanda's manager confirmed this view. The standard assumption that "customers are always right" seems to be adhered to in hospitals (and other sites where goods and services are being sold for profit) in recognition of the power of the consumer on whom hospitals are dependent. Interestingly, profit-oriented corporate principles of "consumer power" have permeated healthcare, supposedly a sector that should be motivated by public good rather than profit. As a result of corporatization, whatever the patients or their relatives demand is catered to, including racial preferences. The status of "maid" is enforced on Amanda (a Black female nurse) by both the patient's relative and her manager.

Amanda felt that there was an assumption that a nurse was there only to serve and that mentality was exaggerated when the nurse happened to be Black. Here we see societal expectations of women even in highly professional roles being expected to serve, unlike what is expected of a doctor or even a male nurse. When combined with expectations of Black people's roles in society, gender becomes conflated with "race." Not only do nurses of colour often not get support from their managers when patients make unfair demands, but they also do not get such support when the demands are coming from doctors. In the latter situation, there is an intimidation factor because doctors tend to be male and of a higher occupational and social status.

Lack of recognition was mentioned by several nurses of colour. Anna, a Black nurse, said:

> I was so confident in my knowledge. I knew that what I said was right and that certain things were the right things to do. They totally contradicted me and sometimes they would go after it is all finished and then they do what I had suggested in the first place. They never gave me credit.

> This surgeon is very controlling to most of us but it seems like he has particular grudge in me. For example, if he is giving instruction to us two nurses — RN [me] and other one RPN — he discusses instruction to the RPN instead of me [even though I was] in charge of care that day since I am the RN. (Asian nurse)

Such a dismissive attitude towards nurses of colour is based on infantilization practices, referred to earlier. More serious consequences can follow from such attitudes, such as formal complaints, not being given leadership roles or being demoted. Part of the dismissive and infantilizing discourse includes the erroneous assumption that nurses of colour are lacking in leadership skills. This assumption is based in age-old racist ideologies about people of colour being incompetent and inferior compared to white people. Even when a nurse of colour is in a leadership role, her authority and competence are likely to be undermined or challenged, as in the case of the Asian nurse quoted above. Colleen talks about a Black nursing supervisor whom she worked with:

> People tended to be much more hostile to her… and they would talk [to] her differently than you would… say somebody in her position. She was their manager… but they were much more hostile to her.

Other issues mentioned by nurses of colour included discrimination in hirings, bumping rights and promotions. Some mentioned isolation, exclusion from decisions, the grapevine and social functions. I would describe these as resulting in the marginalization of these nurses. Some mentioned stereotypical comments being made about them such as "all Blacks have tough skin," "minorities see things different" and that they are "aggressive and confrontational."

Shirley, a Black nurse who filed a grievance for unjust dismissal, was blamed for her own situation because she allegedly had an anger problem. There was no investigation of her supervisor's racism, although her dismissal was found to be unjustified.[2] This is an example of "blaming the victim," a common form of everyday racism.

Political events influence nurses' everyday experiences of racism. One mentioned being asked about her religion following the terrorist attack on the World Trade Centre in September 2001. Another mentioned being subjected to a racial comment following a high profile media story dealing with race. Colleen, a Black nurse, observes:

> Like I have some kind of inside scoop. And, during the O.J. Simpson affair, I seemed to have been singled out as the authoritarian of Black issues, because during the O.J. Simpson trial, I get… consulted on that if, you know, I was keeping tabs on it or not… that's beside the issue. They just assume that somehow, I have sorta the Black hotline.

In response to a related question about whether they had ever felt "put down," insulted or degraded because of race, colour or ethnicity, 40 percent (235 out of 593) replied "yes." Again, cross-tabulating the answers by racial identity, most non-white nurses (79 percent of Black/African Canadians, 83 percent of Asian Canadians, 56 percent of South Asian Canadians, 71 percent of Central/South Americans), and a notable minority of white nurses (23 percent of white/European Canadians) answered "yes" to this question.

All nurses were asked if they had ever witnessed an incident where a nurse was treated differently because of his/her race, colour or ethnicity. Forty-four percent (261 out of 593) replied "yes" to this question, while an almost equal proportion of 43 percent (257 out of 593) replied "no."

THE PERPETRATORS

Nurses were asked who was "putting them down?" The largest proportion (27.3 percent) of "put downs" were experienced at the hands of colleagues, i.e., another nurse. Next in line were patients (23.8 percent), followed by doctors (14.3 percent), managers (12.8 percent) and "others" (8.3 percent). In many instances, nurses of colour are harassed by their managers and colleagues in unison. This is the case in a poisoned environment.

Shirley, a Black nurse mentioned above, worked in a poisoned environment. She was fired for alleged "unprofessional" behaviour towards her supervisors, colleagues and patients. Complaints had been registered by patients and colleagues, and it is noteworthy that all the complaints were from white people even though there were several non-whites working in her unit. Her dismissal had been preceded by a written warning and a suspension. Her supervisor claimed that she felt physically and verbally threatened by Shirley. Shirley claimed that her supervisor was the one who was threatening. Another supervisor of Shirley's also sided against her. Shirley claimed racial harassment, referring to a number of incidents, including repeated night shifts, no choice in holiday timing, racist name-calling and lost pay for being late. None of Shirley's complaints of racism were ever investigated. In my view, Shirley was targeted for exceptionally stringent supervision, monitoring and documentation, typical experiences of everyday racism encountered particularly by strong, outspoken Black nurses who are assertive in their resistance to racism. This is an example of differential management practices based on the principle that differently racialized workers require different types of managerial approaches.

To probe whether there was a relationship between the race/ethnicity of nurses and their perception of whether race/ethnicity/colour affected their relationships with their colleagues, a cross-tabulation was generated between these two aspects. The numbers in Table 5.1 show that significant proportions of non-white nurses, particularly Black (58.1 percent) and Asian Canadians (48.3 percent), perceived that their race/ethnicity/colour affected their relationships with their colleagues.[3] White/European Canadian nurses had the second lowest proportion (17.4 percent) of all groups that had a similar perception, higher only than the "no answer" group, i.e., those who did not identify their ethnic/racial group. Given that nursing is highly ori-

Table 5.1 Did Respondents Feel that Their Race/Ethnicity/Colour Had an Effect on Their Relations with Colleagues?

Racial/Ethnic Group	Yes %	No %	No Answer %
Black/African	58.1	35.5	6.5
Asian	48.3	46.7	5.0
South Asian	27.8	66.7	5.6
Aboriginal/First Nations			
Central/South American	42.9	57.1	
White/European	17.4	78.5	4.2
Other	23.8	72.1	4.1
Not Identified	16.7	58.3	25.0

ented to teamwork, negative relationships with colleagues can have serious consequences in terms of work environment and workload.

To examine whether there was a relationship between the race/ethnicity of nurses and their perceptions of whether their race/ethnicity or colour affected their relationships with patients, a cross-tabulation was generated. Table 5.2 shows that the majority of Black/African Canadian nurses (58.1 percent) felt that their ethnicity/race/colour had an effect on their relationships with patients. Although the majority of other non-white groups of nurses felt that race/ethnicity/colour did not affect their interactions with patients, it is again noteworthy that larger proportions of non-white nurses (35 percent of Asian Canadians, 33.3 percent of South Asian Canadians) compared to white/European Canadian nurses (14.5 percent) felt that race/ethnicity/colour did have an effect on their relationships with patients.

As mentioned before, a question identifying the racial identities of "put downers" was not included in the survey; however, in follow-up interviews this issue was addressed. The harassers were almost always identified as white. Yet, healthcare institutions are ill-prepared to protect nurses from racial harassment from patients.

Daniel, a Black nurse, was physically assaulted by a mentally ill patient who simultaneously hurled racist slurs at him. Although Daniel was asked to leave the room, the racial abuse was not addressed when there was a brief meeting to discuss the incident. On the following day, Daniel, being the charge nurse, had to assign himself to the same abusive patient as there was no one else trained to deal with such a patient. He endured another full day of racial abuse from the patient. This happened with the knowledge of management. Due to the trauma caused by the incidents, Daniel became sick at the end of his shift and stayed home on the third day. Daniel's manager

Table 5.2: Did Respondents Feel that Their Race/Ethnicity/Colour Had an Effect on Their Relations with Their Patients?

Racial/Ethnic Group	Yes %	No %	No Answer %
Black/African	58.1	35.5	6.5
Asian	35.0	58.3	6.7
South Asian	33.3	50.0	16.7
Aboriginal/First Nations			
Central/South American	28.6	57.1	14.3
White/European	14.5	80.1	5.5
Other	24.6	72.1	3.3
Not Identified	16.7	58.3	25.0

responded by calling him several times on the phone and finally sent him a letter directing him to report to work. The manager felt that Daniel could be supported more by his colleagues if he was at work. However, Daniel saw these efforts as further aggravating his stress level. He was not only subjected to racial harassment from a patient, but he was also infantilized and treated differently from other (white) nurses as far as his sick leave provisions were concerned. No other sick nurse had been called by the manager at home and ordered to report back to work. In effect, Daniel's claims of being sick were denied. One can only assume that his manager had decided that Daniel was lying or exaggerating the traumatic effects of being racially harassed and the fact of being ill.

In subsequent grievance arbitration hearings, it was revealed that the hospital had no policy or procedure in place dealing with racial harassment from patients.[4] There was also no known anti-discrimination policy at the hospital. Moreover, the manager had received no education or workshop to deal with such a situation. The only recourses for Daniel were to file for Workers' Compensation and a grievance under his collective agreement, both of which he did. Daniel remained sick for nine days. His Worker's Compensation claim noted that he was traumatized due to the lack of support and intervention from staff and that he suffered from insomnia, lack of concentration and headaches.

HOW THE HARASSMENT AFFECTED THEM

Nurses that I surveyed were asked to comment on how everyday racism affected them (see Table 5.3). The responses confirm what we know anecdotally, that is, racial harassment has serious health effects on its targets. Nurses mentioned emotional effects such as disappointment, anger, feeling degraded, worthlessness, not wanting to return to work, "upset the flow of the day," being silenced, distrustful, sad, disappointed, feeling of resignation, feeling inferior and defensive, thoughts about leaving the profession, being on a "roller coaster" and being "dragged down." Edmonds discusses that all human beings need to feel valued and trusted.

> When a person's authority is constantly questioned and undermined, it will negatively impact self confidence... without a strong sense of ego, it can be difficult to keep going in the face of these obstacles. (2001: 6)

Asha, a South Asian nurse, describes what harassment does to one's self esteem:

> For the longest time there, I thought they were better than me, I think I was made to feel that way.

78

Table 5.3 How the Harassment Affected Respondents*

	Frequency	Percent
Emotionally	202	31.4
Physically	82	13.8
Mentally	134	22.6
Other Ways	102	17.2

* More than one effect was noted by many nurses

Edmonds (2001) describes physical problems that can arise from devaluation; thyroid problems, diabetes and other chronic diseases are often rooted in the constant stress of racism. Feagin (2003: 1) writes that "the major and minor slights of racism can accumulate to a very negative health impact" and that stomach problems, chest pains, hypertension and depression among African Americans are often caused by the suppression of anger and stress caused by racism.

Nurses surveyed for this study reported feeling ill, experiencing a rise in blood pressure and body tension and difficulty sleeping. Under mental health effects, many mentioned being tired, fatigued, exhausted, depressed, distressed and shocked. One person had a nervous breakdown after years of fighting for her rights. Hagey et al.'s (2001) study showed that the physical stress and emotional pain of racism resulted in such symptoms as sudden onset cardiovascular diseases and depression. A few nurses surveyed said that the negative experience made them stronger, more empowered and more willing to fight back.

ACTION TAKEN FOLLOWING HARASSMENT

Some of the reasons given by nurses for not taking any action were that the patients who were harassing were confused, or they were afraid of hurting their job, were caught by surprise and became speechless, were unable to name the problem immediately, did not know their rights, felt that it wouldn't help and, as female nurses, were socialized to be nurturing and kind. Actions taken included talking back assertively, verbalizing their rights to the harasser, threatening to take action, talking to their supervisor, nursing manager, human resource person, ONA representative, filing an incident report and filing grievances. One person said that harassment was a "way of life at the hospital" and that she took action on only "the real bad ones."

RESULT OF ACTIONS FOLLOWING HARASSMENT

Talking back assertively occasionally resulted in positive results as a number of nurses reported that the harassing behaviour stopped or that the harasser

Table 5.4 Result of Actions Taken

	Frequency	Percent
Nothing Happened	87	14.7
Filed a Grievance	4	0.7
Won the Grievance	4	0.7
Person Stopped Put-downs	29	4.9
Other	80	13.5
No Answer	398	65.6

apologized. In more cases, it had no effect. Indeed, eighty-seven nurses who indicated taking some action also reported that their action had no effect on the harassment (see Table 5.4). One can understand why many nurses reported feeling pessimistic about the effectiveness of taking any action at all.

Many of the grievances filed were ongoing.[5] However, survey results indicate that filing a grievance is clearly not a common way of handling racial harassment, with only four (.7 percent) reporting having used this approach. One person said that when she won her grievance, the harassment stopped for a short period of time and then it started up again. Another nurse reported that her tires were slashed. One nurse said that comments were placed on her performance evaluation because she advocated on behalf of minority groups.

Indeed, a review of nineteen arbitration decisions and settlements revealed that only two grievances on the issue of racial discrimination were won by the ONA. All the others were dismissed by the arbitrator due to "lack of evidence." In most of these cases, the arbitrators imply that the racial conflict was generated due to an incorrect perception by the grievor, a communication problem or, in some cases, personality traits of the grievor. The latter demonstrates a "blame the victim" mentality. Clearly, these decisions and judgements are deterrents to nurses taking any action at all following harassment. On the other hand, one nurse commented that following the harassing behaviour, there was:

> Decreased functioning in [her] personal life. After grievance [was] resolved, personal life became very productive. I did feel I won and the institution's behaviour towards me changed and also an internal change in me occurred.

SYSTEMIC RACISM

In my discussion of how racism works, I argued that everyday racism must be viewed within the context of systemic racism involving exclusion, disadvantage or differential treatment of nurses of colour compared to white nurses. A powerful indicator of systemic racism in paid workplaces is racial segregation.

Racial Segregation

The most recent statistical data I could find, from 1991 in Nestel[6] (2000), suggests that while there were significant concentrations of nurses of colour among RNs and RPNs in Ontario and Toronto, they were under-represented among nursing management. While RNs and RPNs of colour made up 17.5 percent of Ontario's nurses, only 7.8 percent (490) of head nurses were people of colour. In Toronto, where nurses of colour made up 33.5 percent of the total nursing population, they accounted for only 18 percent (340) of head nurses.

This indicates racial segregation in nursing, although more up-to-date statistical analysis needs to be undertaken to confirm this fact. Case studies of hospitals point in the same direction. For instance, my study (1994) of the Northwestern General Hospital (NWGH) demonstrated that upper and middle management in that hospital was predominantly white. Even lower level leadership positions, such as that of clinical resource nurse, were predominantly white. Fifty-six percent (56 percent) of nursing staff were identified as "visible minorities," out of which 30 percent were Blacks. This was in contrast to Blacks being only 6.12 percent of the Metro Toronto population in 1986 (the latest figure available at the time of writing). Black nurses were working on the fourth floor and in obstetrics, and were least represented in the intensive care unit (ICU), operating room (OR) and emergency room (ER), the more desirable units to work in. Other visible minority nurses were better represented in OR and ICU.

Caissey (1994) points out the streaming of nurses of colour into low status units such as chronic care, rehabilitation and geriatric care, where advancement is limited and injuries are more apt to happen. This corroborates with other findings (Gustafson 2002; Das Gupta 1996a; DMI and Minors 1994). Thus, it is apparent that racial segregation is both vertical, that is among different classes of female nurses, and it is horizontal, that is among nurses within the same class.

As discussed before, segregation is the result of standard policies, procedures and practices within the systems of employment, including such practices as word-of-mouth hiring and the use of subjective and non-standard methods of "assigning" leadership roles and promoting nurses in general, that result in the exclusion of people of colour from certain areas and their concentration in others.

Word-of-mouth methods of hiring were generally encouraged in the NWGH. The human resource assistant pre-screened candidates, including checking on reference letters. She used personal discretion to decide whether the competition should be broadened or kept among internal candidates. If she felt "iffy" about the latter and if she noticed that applicants had been job-hopping, she would open up the recruitment process. I argue that job hopping may simply reflect employment barriers faced by nurses of colour due to racism rather than their instability as workers (1994). In fact, nurses of colour interviewed for this study spoke about that reality. Job-hopping might also reflect the nature of the labour market rather than the work habits of the worker, as Krahn and Lowe (1988) argue.

Job interviews at the NWGH left a lot of room for subjectivity and bias. Such vague criteria as the "right attitude," "motivation" and "personality types" were used to assess the suitability of applicants. The lack of cross-cultural training of interviewers left them ill-equipped to objectively assess the verbal and non-verbal communication styles of nurses of different ethnic and racial backgrounds. Similar concerns arose around subjective interpretations of criteria on performance appraisal forms and in disciplinary measures.

Gustafson (2002) suggests that the College of Nurses of Ontario (CNO) may encourage immigrant women trained as nurses outside Canada to become UCPs as a way of gaining practical experience and familiarity, thereby preparing for their registration.

To further verify Caissey's argument noted above, nurses surveyed were asked whether race/ethnicity/colour had any effect on where they worked. One-fifth of the nurses (121 out of 593) replied that it did, while almost three-quarters said that it did not. When cross-tabulated with the racial/ethnic identities of nurses, it is clear that non-white nurses reported a connection in larger proportions than did white/European nurses (see Table 5.5). To probe further into how racial segregation occurs systemically, I asked nurses whether race/ethnicity/colour had an effect on their hiring, promotion, training opportunities, accommodation due to disability, sick leave, performance reviews and disciplinary actions. Further, I enquired whether race, ethnicity or colour had any effect on their relationships with colleagues, managers and patients, which would in turn affect their quality of work life and their chances for promotions.

As was true in the Head (1985) study, although most nurses answering my survey had not experienced racism within the employment system, a significant proportion had. For instance, 27 percent responded that race, ethnicity or colour affected their relations with colleagues, and 24 percent noted that the same variables affected their relations with patients. Moreover, when cross-tabulated with race/ethnicity, significantly higher percentages of nurses of colour report the negative impact of their racialization on their workplace experience (see Table 5.6).

It is interesting to note that apart from its impact on promotions, the most racism was reported in relationships with managers, patients and colleagues rather than in ways in which nurses had gained access to hirings, training

Table 5.5 Did Respondents Feel that Their Race/Ethnicity/Colour Had an Effect on Where They Work?

Racial/Ethnic Group	Yes	No	No Answer	Total
Black/African	31 (50%)	23 (37.1%)	8 (12.9%)	62
Asian	28 (46.7%)	30 (50%)	2 (3.3%)	60
South Asian	7 (38.9%)	9 (50%)	2 (11.1%)	18
Aboriginal/First Nations				1
Central/South American	3 (42.9%)	4 (57.1%)		7
White/European	26 (8.4%)	270 (86.8%)	15 (4.8%)	311
Other	25 (20.5%)	95 (77.9%)	2 (1.6%)	122
Not Identified	1 (8.3%)	7 (58.3%)	4 (33.3%)	12
Total	121 (20.4%)	439 (74%)	33 (5.6%)	593

Table 5.6 Percentage Who Reported Their Race/Ethnicity/Colour Had an Effect on Their Employment

	Black	Asian	South Asian	South/Central American	White	Other
Hiring	43.5	50	23.3	42.9	8	13.1
Promotions	56.5	44.4	36.7	28.6	7.1	15.6
Relations with Colleagues	58.1	27.8	48.3	42.9	17.4	23.8
Relations with Managers	54.8	44.4	46.7	28.6	5.8	13.9
Relations with Patients	58.1	33.3	35	28.6	14.5	24.6
Training Opportunities	41.9	33.3	33.3	14.3	3.9	10.7
Performance Reviews	38.7	22.2	20	0	1.3	7.4
Discipline	25.8	0	10	0	2.3	5.7
Accommodation of Disability	6.5	5.6	8.3	14.3	2.6	3.3

opportunities, accommodation due to disability, performance reviews and disciplinary actions. This could be a reflection of the fact that individual behavioural forms of racism are more readily perceived and identified than systemic racism, which deals more with policies, procedures and practices of an institution. While the latter also includes individual behaviours, they are often not directly observed or "justified" by apparently neutral documents and policies.

In the Head (1985) study referred to earlier, dissatisfaction with their employment had been noted by 25.3 percent of Blacks and 8.4 percent of whites, which indicated that "race" was a crucial factor in determining the quality of employment experiences. It was further reported that although the proportions of whites and Blacks applying for promotions were the same, 62.5 percent of the former were successful in being promoted while only 36.4 percent of Blacks were successful. Fifty percent of whites reported positive communication with their supervisors, compared to 34.6 percent of Blacks. About 30 percent of those interviewed reported being harassed by patients. All but one of these people were non-white.

Racism and Hiring

In terms of hiring, 15.8 percent of nurses overall felt that race, ethnicity or colour had an effect on their hiring (see Table 5.7). Cross-tabulated with race, there is a stronger relationship between racial identities of nurses and their experience of racism in hiring situations; more non-white than white nurses felt that their race/ethnicity/colour affected their hiring process.

The nature of racism in hiring varies from one institution to another and for nurses of colour with different lengths of stay in Canada. Amanda, a Black nurse, describes her experience soon after landing in Canada from Britain:

> I just opened the newspaper and saw it and was practically hired until I was told to come down and see them. I was new to the country and obviously at that time, he didn't pick up my accent on the phone and 'cos I had come from England and he maybe thought I was a British nurse and so when I went, he told me that the job was gone… He said, well, you have no Canadian experience… I explained to him it was a job on obstetrics and I said, well, your nurses here train for… maybe a few weeks in obstetrics, I am a trained midwife, don't tell me that that experience doesn't count for anything and he said, oh, it's not Canadian experience… I know that at that time it is because he saw me and who I was, but that was twenty-odd years ago. The job that I'm in… they say they are equal opportunity employers, so I think they have to hire one periodically to show that there is one or two, so when I was hired… I think, I fitted the quota.

Even though Amanda believes that the criterion of "Canadian experience" to exclude the hiring of new immigrant nurses may be passé, others provide a different picture. They suggest that it is still very prevalent as a systemic way in which nurses of colour who are newly arrived in Canada are denied jobs. This seemingly standard criterion disadvantages workers of colour most specifically. The requirement of "Canadian experience" does not

Table 5.7 Did Respondents Feel that Their Race/Ethnicity/Colour Had an Effect on Their Hiring?

Racial/Ethnic Group	Yes	No	No Answer	Total
Black/African	27 (43.5%)	33 (53.2%)	2 (3.2%)	62
Asian	14 (23.3%)	43 (71.7%)	3 (5%)	60
South Asian	9 (50%)	8 (44.4%)	1 (5.6%)	18
Aboriginal/First Nations				1
Central/South American	3 (42.9%)	4 (57.1%)		7
White/European	25 (8%)	277 (89.1%)	9 (2.9%)	311
Other	16 (13.1%)	101 (82.8%)	5 (4.1%)	122
Not Identified		9 (75%)	3 (25%)	12
Total	94 (15.9%)	476 (80.3%)	23 (3.9%)	593

on the face of it contain any race-related discourse. Instead, it tends to privilege nurses who have been trained and working in Canada over newcomer nurses of any ethnic background. The implication of this requirement is that those who have been trained and employed in Canada have something that is lacking in those who have not. As discussed previously, a value judgement is made that Canadian training and employing institutions are superior to those outside Canada. Considering that most newcomers to Canada today are people of colour and that a Canadian is associated in common-sensical terms with whiteness, the requirement of Canadian experience takes on a racialized tone. We can see how a discourse of citizenship or nationalism hides the discourse of race and has the result of disadvantaging newcomer nurses of colour most of all.

The phenomenon of tokenism, referred to by Amanda, is another indicator of systemic racism. It ensures that the employing organization is doing only the bare minimum in terms of representation of people of colour in the workforce. However, it does not ensure that the person of colour thus hired will feel comfortable enough to remain in the job, or that she will have any power or authority in it. Melissa, a Black nurse, was awarded the position of senior public health nurse following her grievance for being denied a promotion despite the fact that she was more qualified than her colleagues. However, she was not given the responsibilities normally assigned to her position. To escape such peculiar situations, many tokenized individuals will eventually move on to other jobs.

Today, after many years of living in Canada, Amanda faces obstacles in her efforts to gain a management position.

I have developed and worked hard at developing and I don't feel that they

Table 5.8 Did Respondents Feel that Their Race/Ethnicity/Colour Had an Effect on Their Relations with Their Manager?

Racial/Ethnic Group	Yes	No	No Answer	Total
Black/African	34 (54.8%)	22 (35.5%)	6 (9.7%)	62
Asian	28 (46.7%)	30 (50%)	2 (3.3%)	60
South Asian	8 (44.4%)	9 (50%)	1 (5.6%)	18
Aboriginal/First Nations				1
Central/South American	2 (28.6%)	5 (71.4%)		7
White/European	18 (5.1%)	279 (89.7%)	14 (4.5%)	311
Other	17 (13.9%)	100 (82%)	5 (4.1%)	122
Not Identified	1 (8.3%)	8 (66.7%)	3 (25%)	12
Total	109 (18.4%)	453 (76.4%)	31 (5.2%)	593

> are being tapped into… and like I said I consistently see people who have two years' nursing experience… and they get the job. So, what else could there be? It's funny, I was saying to somebody… to my manager today, I said the only thing I can come up with is that they can say, well, you know what, I am not an organizational fit. And, that would mean that, well, looking at their organization and looking at their management team and all that, yes, I don't fit because they are mostly all white.

Amanda is very perceptive in identifying how subtle practices, including using subjective and vague criteria such as "organizational fit," are often used to weed out candidates from jobs. Such practices, which are examples of systemic racism, usually result in the reproduction of white management within organizations. Nurses of different statuses become divided along racial lines.

I probed further on whether race, ethnicity or colour had an effect on nurses' relationships with their managers. Cross-tabulations produced the results noted in Table 5.8. Most (54.8 percent) Black/African Canadian nurses said that their race/ethnicity/colour affected their relationship with their manager, and the same was true for sizeable proportions of Asian Canadian nurses (46.7 percent) and South Asian Canadian nurses (44.4 percent). Amanda explains her perception of her manager's relationship with her:

> I think deep down some are fairly… intimidated by me, because I don't hold back what I want to say to them because I think they need to hear… Right now, I have a problem where if I go for a job and put in references, I don't know who to put because none of them really know me… what will it be based on? Maybe my personality, that… I am very confrontational, you know, so it's hard… because you see I'm not a timid person… So, for the managers they have difficulty with that and like even my own manager.

> She has less experience than me. She has been in the department less time than me. She has less qualifications than me, but she is my manager because she is blonde.

Amanda's confidence, leadership qualities, experience and education make her an ideal candidate for management. However, she has not had an opportunity to prove her potential. Instead, her positive qualities position her as a threat to her manager and her colleagues.

This section provides information on how racial segregation is being reproduced within healthcare settings through systemically racist policies and practices around recruitment and placement. Moreover, Amanda's experience begins to address how one's relationship with one's manager has a direct effect on one's chances for good references and promotion. The next section develops these issues further.

Racism and Promotions

Ninety-seven (18 percent) nurses in the overall survey felt that race, ethnicity or colour had an effect on their access to promotions. Cross tabulated with race/ethnicity, the patterns in Table 5.9 emerge. There is a strong relationship between race/ethnicity of nurses and whether they perceive that promotions in nursing were influenced by race/ethnicity/colour. Overall, 28.6 to 56.5 percent of non-white groups answered affirmatively to this question, but only 7.1 percent of white/European Canadian nurses did.

Colleen, a Black nurse on her way to completing a master's degree, talks about the discouragement that she faced in applying for a nurse educator position:

> Well, I remember one time there was a position coming up and it had to do with who was informed. I know that when they were looking for this position, the person had to have, or at least be well on the way into a master's degree… so there was limitation on my part because… I was accepted, but I had not begun one course yet. So I was quite surprised to find out that not only did they hire an educator without a master's degree or not even enrolled in a master's degree… but one with a baccalaureate and three years' experience when they were looking for someone with five to seven years' experience.

Apart from the fact that she had not been informed fully about the position, Colleen talks about how a white nurse with less than the advertised educational requirements and experience was hired. Colleen, with more appropriate educational credentials, was not encouraged to apply. In the following anecdote, she talks further about the lack of mentoring experienced by nurses of colour and the effects of that on their work lives.

> I think that a person of colour probably gonna have to… probably will have

Table 5.9 Did Respondents Feel that Their Race/Ethnicity/Colour Had an Effect on Their Promotion?

Racial/Ethnic Group	Yes	No	No Answer	Total
Black/African	35 (56.5%)	20 (32.3%)	7 (11.3%)	62
Asian	22 (36.7%)	30 (50%)	8 (13.3%)	60
South Asian	8 (44.4%)	7 (38.9%)	3 (16.7%)	18
Aboriginal/First Nations				1
Central/South American	2 (28.6%)	5 (71.4%)		7
White/European	22 (7.1%)	272 (87.5%)	17 (5.5%)	311
Other	19 (15.6%)	94 (77%)	9 (7.4%)	122
Not Indicated	1 (8.3%)	8 (66.7%)	3 (25%)	12
Total	109 (18.4%)	437 (73.7%)	47 (7.9%)	593

a hard time getting tenure in any organization, if they are not informed or mentored. And if they want to say, be a manager somewhere, say a nursing manager on a unit and they are not getting the mentorship to be there, then they will go somewhere else because the idea is to be a manager… And a lot of my colleagues, who may be of colour, tend to move around… I don't think my white counterparts have moved around or needed to move and change jobs as often over the years… I've often seen that the white nurses get to stay where they are and even if they are… trying to move up the ladder in any way, there's always been in a position or a position created or encouragement to stay there and get mentored into another position… as they are moving their way and getting their experience… I wouldn't be surprised if I finish my PhD, then end up in the States.

Asha, a South Asian nurse, talked about how she was doing the work of a charge nurse but was never formally given that title.

I was doing charge position and sort of not officially… And I was taking the initiative to do other things, so I just asking to make it more official… I asked for an appointment to meet with her… nope, didn't even get an appointment.

Anna, a Black nurse, reported that her head nurse consistently put her "at the bottom of her list" for the "in charge person" despite the fact that she was the most educated and most experienced nurse in the unit. Many similar stories were found in the course of this research.

The level of education one has is a predictor of where one will practise nursing and also whether one will experience upward mobility or not. Perhaps this is the reason why many nurses of colour are studying part-time for graduate degrees. Many are encountering barriers within the education system at the same time as trying to juggle work life and, in most cases, family life. To begin with, nursing education in particular and education in general is less available to those who are financially disadvantaged, including new immigrants and people of colour. New immigrants experience the added barrier of devaluation of their degrees and experiences prior to immigration.

Racism and Training Opportunities

A majority of the nurses surveyed did not answer a question regarding whether they were satisfied with the way their foreign education was assessed. Perhaps this was because the sample of respondents was not representative of nurses who came with nursing education from outside Canada. This raises a number of methodological questions. Does the low response indicate that foreign trained nurses are under-represented within the ONA? Or, perhaps that they simply did not respond to the survey? Of those who answered the question (20.2 percent), 15.5 percent reported that they were satisfied.

Systemic racism in the assessment of nursing qualifications from outside Canada was made abundantly clear during the arbitral hearings of two ONA grievances involving the Clarke Institute in Toronto.[7] Two Black nurses had been placed on a salary grid with no recognition of their nursing experience outside Canada. One of them had been told that such experience was not "normally" recognized. This policy remained until the early 1990s, when a nursing shortage and the desire to attract and retain skilled nurses prompted the hospital to examine its accreditation policy.

During the arbitration hearings, it was revealed that the hospital had a practice prior to that time of giving credit to "out of country" experience only if it was from the U.K., U.S. or another Canadian province. This policy was patterned after the Ontario College of Nurses' standards for accepting foreign credentials. Even the ONA initially was reluctant to pursue this grievance because it did not want to jeopardize its relationship with the hospital and to question the longstanding policy on accreditation.

It was also revealed that the Clarke Institute made exceptions for some foreign-born nurses who were white, but that Black nurses from the "in" countries were not given recognition. For instance, a Black nurse with over twenty years of nursing experience from England was denied any credit when she was hired. The final decision of the arbitrator mentioned sloppy personnel practices, inconsistencies and mistakes. Policies were often vague and not written down. Placement on the salary grid depended on who did the processing, and policies were applied liberally to the advantage of white nurses whereas they were strictly followed to the disadvantage of Black nurses. Even after the hospital decided to give credit for all out-of-country experience, it was done in an inconsistent manner. The process depended on the person making the claim. The board of arbitration unanimously held that the Clarke Institute policy was racially discriminatory and ruled that each of the grievors be paid $6,000 for mental anguish and losses. Unfortunately, salary adjustments for the grievors were not ordered retroactively to the date of their hiring and the ONA's request for a review of payments to all nurses in that hospital with foreign qualifications was denied.

Nowhere was systemic racism against foreign trained nurses more evident than in the situation of graduate nurses[8] in Ontario precipitated by the *Regulated Health Professions Act* in 1994, a situation that prompted the ONA to request the OHRC to initiate a complaint against the College of Nurses of Ontario on the basis of disability, race and ethnic origin (MacDonald 1995). The Act for the first time included graduate nurses within the jurisdiction of the CNO, which meant that they would have to be registered with the CNO. The CNO allowed for provisional registration for those graduate nurses who were employed in nursing, restricted them from performing controlled acts even on an order and required them to pass the Canadian Nursing Association Testing Services (CNATS) exam within a period of three years in order to gain full registration and in that way continue with their duties. Failing that, they would not be registered and thus would have to be demoted to nurse's aides or orderlies or terminated from employment. The latter was highly likely since the environment as described earlier was marked by fiscal crises and a restriction on the performance of controlled acts would render them unqualified for their jobs. In fact, twenty-two graduate nurses at St. Joseph's Health Centre in Toronto were laid off on January 1, 1995, for failing to have provisional registration, either due to not writing the CNATS exam or not being able to pass it.

There were approximately 200 graduate nurses affected, most of whom were older, experienced women of colour, trained as nurses outside Canada. Many of them had been brought into Canada during a period of nursing shortage during the 1960s and 1970s and therefore had been working for decades with the same employer with excellent performance appraisals.

In 1981, when the ONA and the Ontario Hospital Association signed an agreement for all non-registered nurses or nursing assistants to become registered within twenty-four months, these graduate nurses were "grandparented" on condition that if they changed employment, they would also have to become registered within the same period of time.

When the CNO announced the requirement for passing the CNATS exam as a condition for graduate nurses, it is noteworthy that it went against the CNO staff recommendation, which was to extend the existing grandparent clause. The Minister of Health on two occasions wrote letters urging the CNO to delete the three-year time limitation imposed on graduate nurses and subsequently suggested that they should be given ten years to fulfill that condition. These requests were rejected by the CNO on the pretext of safeguarding the public interest. The OHRC decided to pursue the complaint against the CNO as well as the Ministry of Health, which was deemed to have the power to intervene in the situation but had not done so (OHRC 1997).

The ONA argued also that the CNATS exam requirement was an invalid ground for assessing the competency of nurses as the test was culturally biased and covered a far wider ground than was relevant for graduate nurses (MacDonald 1995). It was pointed out that the CNO itself recognized this fact and that the new requirement for nurses, which would be in effect in 1997, would not include writing the exam. Instead, it would provide a choice to nurses of four options: performance appraisals, formal education, professional improvement or a professional portfolio (MacDonald 1995). Thus, the graduate nurses were the only group that were singled out and required by the CNO to write the exam. The ONA reported that the CNO was denying registration to some nurses who were registered in Quebec and the U.S. Also, nurses who were not registered with the CNO were being denied access into education programs unless they wrote the CNATS exam (MacDonald 1995).

That the CNO used its discretion on this issue is demonstrated by the fact that when certain employers appealed for graduate nurses to continue with restricted duties, the CNO obliged them. It also waived the exam requirement for seven individuals who were within five years of retirement; yet it could not make accommodations for the majority of graduate nurses. In fact, the CNO has grandparented nurses in the past. For instance, nurses aides were registered as registered nursing assistants and nurses trained in the U.K. and U.S. were registered as nurses following the completion of a refresher course. It appears that the CNO had differential standards of public safety regarding nurses trained in the U.S. and U.K. than those trained in the Philippines and the Caribbean.

Sadly, in November 2001, the ONA discovered during a routine call to the OHRC that the Commission had withdrawn its complaint on March 31, 2000, for an unknown and unstated reason. As Barb Wahl, ONA Provincial President at the time, stated "regretfully, the Commission has failed them and lost credibility in the process" (Wahl 2002). By their inaction, both the Ministry of Health and Long Term Care as well as the OHRC have been complicit in systemic racism against the graduate nurses.

A few nurses interviewed for this study talked about their dissatisfaction with the credential recognition system. For example, Amanda, an experienced nurse from England, describes her educational experience upon arriving in Canada:

> My training [had been for] four years and when I came here, they told me I had… I did not have enough hours in psychiatry and I had to go to Centennial College where they concocted this little course… for graduate nurses trained outside Canada… and that was the worst experience of my life… I was never so angry… they were all women of colour and most of

us were trained in England… some were trained in the Caribbean… and when I went to the hospital, I can remember being asked to watch them, watch my first delivery and I stood there and being trained and worked as a midwife… that was so hard for me, watching an intern do delivery and didn't even know what he was doing… and when I went on the postpartum floor and was asked to diaper and feed a baby … I felt very demoralized in terms of the four years' training plus working in a teaching hospital and teaching midwifery and teaching nursing before I came to this country, and I had to go back to the classroom and go to X hospital and where I couldn't even touch an I.V.… I think it had run through and the patient asked… and my colleague turned it off and oh, she was totally told off, you're not to touch anything. We were really treated worse than first year nursing students and at the end of it, when I was being evaluated, I remember her comment was that, I seemed angry… and I said… if you were in my situation, you'd be more than angry.

After being hired in a nursing position, Amanda started undergraduate studies and she experienced a lack of support from her manager and colleagues in doing this. At the time, she was the only person of colour in her unit. Amanda was told that working full-time, studying part-time and having a child was a problem. She was told that she was doing too much, although there were no complaints about her work performance. Ultimately, she had to quit that job since her study schedule would not be accommodated by her manager. In fact, she was labelled as "inflexible" when she informed her manager that she could not work during her scheduled shift as she had to go to school at that time. In her next job, Amanda was able to finish her undergraduate degree because another nurse, who was Black, agreed to switch shifts with her regularly in order to enable her to attend school.

To examine whether training opportunities were equally accessible to nurses of all ethnicities and racial groups, I included a question in the survey on whether they felt that their race/ethnicity/colour had an effect on training opportunities in nursing. Cross-tabulating the responses by the racial/ethnic identities of nurse respondents shows that most nurses, including white and non-white nurses, felt that race/ethnicity/colour had no effect on training opportunities (see Table 5.10). However, as was revealed by other cross-tabulations, more non-white nurses reported that their race/ethnicity/colour had an effect on their training opportunities. Significant minorities of Black Canadian nurses (41.9 percent), Asian Canadian nurses (33.3 percent) and South Asian Canadian nurses (33.3 percent) made such a report, while only 3.9 percent of white/European Canadian nurses did so.

Two other areas of manager-staff nurse relations were examined, namely performance appraisals and disciplinary actions, both of which have a direct relationship to promotional opportunities. Table 5.11 demonstrates that more nurses of colour (38.7 percent of Black/African Canadians, 22.2 percent of

Table 5.10 Did Respondents Feel that Their Race/Ethnicity/Colour Had an Effect on Their Training Opportunities?

Racial/Ethnic Group	Yes	No	No Answer	Total
Black/African	26 (41.9%)	30 (48.4%)	6 (9.7%)	62
Asian	20 (33.3%)	36 (60%)	4 (6.7%)	60
South Asian	6 (33.3%)	9 (50%)	3 (16.7%)	18
Aboriginal/First Nations				1
Central/South American	1 (14.3%)	6 (85.7%)		7
White/European	12 (3.9%)	283 (91%)	16 (5.1%)	311
Other	13 (10.7%)	105 (86.1%)	4 (3.3%)	122
No Answer	2 (16.7%)	7 (58.3%)	3 (25%)	12
Total	80 (13.5%)	477 (80.4%)	36 (6.1%)	593

Table 5.11 Did Respondents Feel that Their Race/Ethnicity/Colour Had an Effect on Their Performance Reviews?

Racial/Ethnic Group	Yes	No	No Answer	Total
Black/African	24 (38.7%)	32 (51.6%)	6 (9.7%)	62
Asian	12 (20%)	47 (78.3%)	1 (1.7%)	60
South Asian	4 (22.2%)	11 (61.1%)	3 (16.7%)	18
Aboriginal/First Nations				1
Central/South American		7		7
White/European	4 (1.3%)	288 (92.6%)	19 (6.1%)	311
Other	9 (7.4%)	107 (87.7%)	6 (4.9%)	122
Not Indicated	1 (8.3%)	8 (66.7%)	3 (25%)	12
Total	54 (9.1%)	501 (84.5%)	38 (6.4%)	593

South Asian Canadians and 20 percent of Asian Canadians) felt that their race/ethnicity/colour has an effect on the way their workplace performance is reviewed compared to only 1 percent of white/European Canadians.

Racism and Disciplinary Procedures

Shirley, a Black nurse, filed a grievance after being fired following a written warning and a suspension. Although she won her grievance and was reinstated in her job, the arbitrator noted that she had a problem with angry outbursts.[9] When Shirley denied this problem, saying that her supervisor's racism contributed to her outburst, the arbitrator stated that she was leaning towards not reinstating her even though her dismissal was unjustified. In the end, she was reinstated simply because the unit she had the conflicts with had been transferred to another hospital.

An important point related to the disciplinary measures taken against Shirley is the different level of tolerance for errors made by nurses of colour. The ONA argued that Shirley was disciplined for making certain errors in documenting for which other (white) nurses would not be disciplined. This is unfortunately a common occurrence, which was also noted in the Northwestern General Hospital and other cases.

Sybil, a senior nurse, was terminated because of alleged chronic absenteeism. This was a complex case in which her absenteeism was caused by the denial of work accommodation entitled to her due to multiple disabilities partially caused by a workplace injury. When she was terminated, she had been suffering from bronchitis. Prior to this incident, she had been on modified work due to a recent injury. While she was sick with bronchitis, her employer decided to eliminate her modified work program despite the fact that she intended to return to work after recovering from her bronchitis. This case demonstrates not only unjust dismissal but also failure to accommodate disabilities.

In Sybil's story, we see how different discourses intersected, namely race, disability, class and gender. As stated before, several authors (Hill-Collins 1990; Davis 1981; Brand 1999) have written about racialized gendered notions that developed in the context of slavery in the United States. These notions position Black women as physically strong, able to withstand inhuman conditions. Moreover, this strength was not usually seen as a positive attribute, but rather as brutish and representing the nullification of her womanhood and a denial of her femininity. Sybil's injury at work is worth reflecting on. Nursing is a very injury-prone occupation as the job requires a great deal of lifting and other physical work. As described before, it has been reported that Black women are allocated the most physically demanding jobs and units in healthcare settings (Das Gupta 1996a, 1996b). Despite Sybil's work-related injury and her chronic bronchitis, her workplace accommodation was eliminated. Presumably, a decision had been made by her superiors that she was not disabled any more or that she should be able to carry on regular nursing activities despite her disability. It seems that demands from her for accommodation were judged to be exaggerated and dishonest. Propensity to immorality is also a part of anti-Black racist ideology and this played into the removal of Sybil's work modification. The result of this denial was chronic absenteeism and being unable to perform her duties. This provided the managerial rationale for disciplinary measures through her dismissal. Sybil won her grievance and was reinstated.[10]

To probe the question of disciplinary procedures and its link with racism, I asked nurses if their race/ethnicity/colour had an effect on any disciplinary action to which they may have been subjected (see Table 5.12). Similar to

Table 5.12 Did Respondents Feel that Their Race/Ethnicity/Colour Had an Effect on Any Disciplinary Action?

Racial/Ethnic Group	Yes	No	No Answer	Total
Black/African	16 (25.8%)	38 (61.3%)	9 (12.9%)	62
Asian	6 (10%)	44 (73.3%)	10 (16.7%)	60
South Asian		16 (88.9%)	2 (11.1%)	18
Aboriginal/First Nations				1
Central/South American		7 (100%)		7
White/European	7 (2.3%)	283 (91%)	21 (6.8%)	311
Other	7 (5.7%)	109 (89.3%)	6 (4.9%)	122
No Answer	1 (8.3%)	8 (66.7%)	3 (25%)	12
Total	37 (6.2%)	506 (85.3%)	50 (8.4%)	593

trends in previous sections, 25.8 percent of Black/African Canadians and 10.0 percent of Asian Canadians compared to 2 percent of white/European Canadians felt such an effect. In contrast to earlier trends, no South Asian Canadians or Central/South American Canadians felt the same way. These patterns indicate that different ethnic groupings of nurses have different workplace experiences where disciplinary procedures are concerned.

Racism in Accommodation of Disabilities

The case of Sybil illustrates the intersection of racism, sexism and ableism. Her story and similar stories related by nurses of colour prompted me to include a question on their access to disability accommodation (see Table 5.13). In general, there were small proportions of each ethnic/racial group who said that their race/ethnicity/colour had an effect on their access to accommodation due to disability. However, there were more non-white nurses compared to white/European Canadians who agreed that there was a relationship.

Priya, a South Asian nurse who injured her back at work, related experiences that illustrate the lack of accommodation of her disabilities. She applied for promotions several times and never succeeded despite the fact that she was the nurse in charge. On one occasion, she asked her manager why she did not get a certain position despite her seniority. The manager told her that it was because she was disabled.

In another hospital, after a painful back surgery, Priya was advised to take physiotherapy full-time rather then part-time, after which she would be placed in an appropriate unit. Upon her return from full-time physiotherapy, she was told that there was no place for her. Instead, she was sent for re-training to be a laboratory technician. Needless to say, she was devastated, but she

Table 5.13 Did Respondents Feel that Their Race/Ethnicity/Colour Had an Effect on Their Access to Accommodation due to Disability?

Racial/Ethnic Group	Yes	No	No Answer	Total
Black/African	4 (6.5%)	38 (61.3%)	20 (32.3%)	62
Asian	5 (8.3%)	40 (66.7%)	15 (25%)	60
South Asian	1 (5.6%)	12 (66.7%)	5 (27.8%)	18
Aboriginal/First Nations				1
Central/South American	1 (14.3%)	3 (42.9%)	3 (42.9%)	7
White/European	8 (2.6%)	245 (78.8%)	58 (18.6%)	311
Other	4 (3.3%)	103 (84.4%)	15 (12.3%)	122
Not Indicated	1 (8.3%)	7 (58.3%)	5 (41.7%)	12
Total	23 (3.9%)	449 (75.7%)	121 (20.4%)	593

had no other choice.

Novelette, a Black nurse whose doctor requested light duties following her pregnancy, was not granted this accommodation. Presumably her disability was not believed by her employer. In time, she became very ill as a result of a series of incidents that she alleged constituted harassment. However, she was denied sick leave. Her employer felt that she was exaggerating her symptoms. After several months of deliberation, she was granted partial sick pay although she had to provide a doctor's certificate for every two-week period, which was not customary for other workers. Novelette's own doctor's reports were disregarded and her employer wanted a psychiatric report as to whether she was fit to return to work.[11]

In each of these cases, we see how nurses of colour who were disabled and needed workplace accommodation were denied it on the basis of certain assumptions. The first assumption was that their disability was either exaggerated or a figment of their imagination. We see this clearly in the cases of Sybil and Novelette. Novelette's having to provide a doctor's note every two weeks for partial sick payment also smacked of infantilization. The second assumption was that these disabled nurses of colour were incompetent. Priya was judged to be unfit for promotion; Sybil was unable to perform her job because of the lack of accommodation; and Novelette was made sick because of the denial of her disability. Not only was Novelette disbelieved regarding her need for accommodation, but her doctor was also disbelieved. Presumably, both she and her doctor were assumed to "have cooked up this scheme" to drain the system, just as Sybil had been disbelieved. They were deemed to be dishonest and corrupt.

Racism in Granting Sick Leave

Following from Novelette's experience, I asked nurses if their race/ethnicity/colour had any effect as far as sick leave provisions were concerned (see Table 5.14). As in other areas, nurses of colour in higher proportions indicated that their race/ethnicity/colour had an effect on their access to sick leave. They range from 22.2 percent of South Asian Canadians to 10.0 percent of Asian Canadians. On the other hand, only 2.9 percent of white/European Canadians gave the same indication.

Apart from information that was formally asked of nurses, either through the survey or direct interviews, many nurses jotted down additional comments in spaces that were provided on the questionnaire. An analysis of these comments revealed interesting ideas about race and racism, both explicitly and implicitly. These are explored in the next chapter.

Table 5.14 Did Respondents Feel that Their Race/Ethnicity/Colour Had an Effect on Their Sick Leave?

Racial/Ethnic Group	Yes	No	No Answer	Total
Black/African	13 (21%)	43 (69.4%)	6 (9.7%)	62
Asian	6 (10%)	48 (80%)	6 (10%)	60
South Asian	4 (22.2%)	12 (66.7%)	2 (11.1%)	18
Aboriginal/First Nations				1
Central/South American	1 (14.3%)	6 (85.7%)		7
White/European	9 (2.9%)	280 (90%)	22 (7.1%)	311
Other	5 (4.1%)	112 (91.8%)	5 (4.1%)	122
Not Indicated	1 (8.3%)	8 (66.7%)	3 (25%)	12
Total	39 (6.6%)	510 (86%)	44 (7.4 %)	593

NOTES

1. Although I did not ask them about the race or ethnicity of the patient in the survey, comments made on the survey and the interviews revealed that most of these patients were white, some from non-English backgrounds.
2. See *St. Michael's Hospital v. Ontario Nurses' Association*, unreported decision of I.G. Thorne dated June 20, 1994.
3. Note that the sole Aboriginal nurse's answers are not being reported here to maintain his/her anonymity and confidentiality.
4. See *Clarke Institute of Psychiatry v. Ontario Nurses' Association*, unreported decision of Belinda Kirkwood dated April 12, 1996.
5. Many nurses who had ongoing grievances answered "other" on the survey.
6. Statistical data were not readily available on ethnic/racial breakdowns in nursing. Nestel (2000) was the only author who made reference to some actual figures. However, the figures are from 1991. Some advocacy effort needs to be undertaken

for the collection of information based on racial/ethnic identities just as it is done on gender

7. See *Re Clarke Institute of Psychiatry v. Ontario Nurses' Association* 95 LAC (4th) 155 (2001).

8. Graduate nurses were immigrant nurses brought into Canada to fill nursing shortages. They were not registered nurses because they had not been tested by the College of Nurses and not given their licence. However, they had been allowed to practise restricted duties.

9. See *St. Michael's Hospital v. Ontario Nurses' Association*, unreported decision of I.G. Thorne dated June 20, 1994.

10. See *Hamilton Civics Hospital v. Ontario Nurses' Association*, unreported decision of R. Verity dated October 12, 1995.

11. See *Northwestern General Hospital v. Ontario Nurses' Association*, unreported decision of D. Starkman dated July 2, 1993.

6. EXPLORING "RACE" AND RACISM AT WORK
Deconstructing What Was Said

The survey conducted for this study included several places where respondents could write brief comments or elaborate on their answers. Although many nurses did not write anything in these spaces, some did, and I was quite taken aback by how candid some of these comments were. Perhaps the anonymity of the survey provoked them to vent some of their deep-seated yet unarticulated thoughts on racism at work. The comments were by and large very revealing and helped me to make sense of how they responded overall to the questions.[1] Most nurses of colour elaborated on their everyday as well as more systemic experiences of racism. Many of these were excerpted and quoted in the last chapter. Most white nurses who wrote commented on such things as reverse racism, denial of racism or playing the "race" card. A few wrote about their own experiences of discrimination as ethnic minorities. This chapter is a discussion of these comments. Many of these comments deal with popular discourses of racism, and their hidden assumptions, worldviews and implications are made explicit through their deconstruction.

ETHNOCENTRISM AND RACIALIZATION

A small number of white nurses felt discriminated against due to their ethnicity, which was racialized by members of the dominant ethnic group. They were categorized as "different" from the norm due to their non-dominant language status, their perceived immigration status and their class. In turn, they were subjected to "put downs" and discriminated against because they were stereotyped as being inferior. For instance, a French-Canadian nurse felt uncomfortable and "put down" whenever she spoke in French. Makropoulos (2004) has discussed the historical racialization of Frenchness vis-à-vis English Canadians, with the most blatant example being the deportation of over 10,000 Acadians, who refused to swear an oath of allegiance to the British Crown in 1755. Even as recently as the 1940s and 1950s, there were occasions of Franco-Ontarians being told to "speak white," meaning speak English. What is revealed here is the social construction of "white" and "non-white" in particular social and political contexts. Not only are racial meanings shifting over time and place, but they are also relational, i.e., in terms of who the "others" are.

A Jewish nurse talked about "put down" comments from colleagues because of her religion. A white nurse of minority ethnicity said

[She was] routinely, referred to as "immigrant"… In an interview was stated "we have another one of you"… Accused of harassment when I defended myself. (white nurse)

As discussed earlier, the term "immigrant" in Canada is a code for "non-white." Whiteness is common-sensically associated with being "Canadian," and anyone who is not white risks the chance of being labelled as an "outsider" or "an immigrant." Thus, such identity labels are highly racialized. In addition, racialization is affected by one's class background and ethnic attributes. Khayatt (1994), originally from Egypt, discusses her own experience of being denied the label "immigrant" by a cleaner, a woman of Southern European origin, because the former came from an upper-class background who was an academic in Canada and spoke English and French fluently. In contrast, the cleaner was working class and non-English speaking. Chances are that the white nurse quoted above was referred to as "immigrant" because of her "accent." Class, linguistic and regional origins are also used to label people as racialized "others," as in the case of the nurse below:

> It was directly stated that because I was from European descent and daughter of a farmer that I could not possibly be knowledgeable. I married an Anglophone with a British name — whose surname I chose to use, so most of the put-downs stopped — Even today after forty years of nursing when people, i.e., co-workers, find out that I am the daughter of a Ukrainian farmer (who could not read or write English) are amazed that I became an RN and subsequently achieved two university degrees and held management/ teaching positions. (white nurse)

> During war in Yugoslavia many would ask what region I was from if they saw my last name — and treated me differently. I was glad when my last name changed when I got married. (white nurse)

It is interesting how the excerpts above reveal a process of othering, whereby apparently white nurses were discriminated against and subjected to everyday classism and racialization by other white nurses, who perceived them as "different" and "inferior." These narratives reveal the connection between "race" and ethnicity and how religion, language, accent and ethnicity, in addition to "race," are implicated in the construction of whiteness. Non-dominant language, accent, religion or ethnic origin can render a person as "not quite white." These statements by nurses reveal experiences of being infantilized and scapegoated similar to what nurses of colour experience, although on a much smaller scale.

However, the way in which nurses of colour experience racism goes beyond the everyday forms. They experience systemic policies and procedures that have the effect of segregating them into less desirable areas of nursing. There was no evidence in my study of systemic racism for white women of minority ethnic backgrounds or whose first language was not English. Moreover, for these racialized white women, their difference from the Anglo mainstream culture diminishes with time, as they assimilate, learn the English language and/or change their names by marrying Anglo men. Makropoulos (2004) talks about how cultural assimilation, particularly linguistic assimilation, became an official colonial policy aimed at "whitening" French-Canadians. Now, French is an official language of Canada, since the *Official Languages Act* of 1969, and it thus enjoys a status equal to that of English, a position not enjoyed by any other language. Having been included in the exclusive club, it seems also that French Canadians have been marked as "officially white," so much so that French-Canadians of colour remain marginalized as not quite French, thus indicating that Frenchness is represented as whiteness in the dominant French Canadian psyche. Nurses of colour have no escape routes from racism. Their skin colour and other physical markers remain with them over time and no amount of cultural assimilation reduces the racism they face. As in the case of French-Canadians, European Jews and Ukrainians, who were all racialized in earlier periods in Canada in relation to English-Canadians, are now seen as white in relation to those with dark skin.

DENIAL OF RACISM

In addition to instances of racialization and racism faced by certain white nurses, there was a wide variety of racist discourses expressed by white nurses and a small number of nurses of colour that denied the existence of racism. Some nurses of colour said that they did not experience or witness racism. There is an articulation of a "blame the victim" argument in the following excerpts:

> I have not witnessed any incidents in which race, colour or ethnicity has played a role in how nurses are treated. I believe how a nurse acts professionally will determine how others will respond. In other words, a lack of professionalism on the nurse's part may lead to a negative perception or response from others. (white nurse)

> I feel there are minority persons who are too sensitive about their own differences and therefore view racism to a greater extent. If a person has high self confidence and good work ethics that person will be less likely to be discriminated against d/t greater respect from larger group of co-workers. (Asian nurse)

Even though this nurse of colour blames the victim and denies the prevalence of racism, she reported elsewhere on her survey that she had felt uncomfortable because of her race/colour/ethnicity when a co-worker spoke to her, to another colleague and to patients who did not speak English well in a verbally demeaning way.

Others simply choose to condone racism from people who are unwell because they rationalize it as "being confused" or "being sick."

> I have been called different names due to me being dark by confused elderly people at the hospital. It has hurt me but I felt they are confused. (S. Asian nurse)

When I read the above comment, I wondered whether this was a way of accommodating abusive behaviour in their caregiving roles or is it something that women are socialized to do? Alternatively, it could be a way of coping with racism in a setting where the perpetrator is in a vulnerable state — sick, elderly or even dying — where anti-racism policies are non-existent or non-functional.

BLAMING THE VICTIM

A denial of racism is usually accompanied with the discourse of blaming the victim of racism as in the excerpts above where nurses of colour who claim to be victims of racism are described as "unprofessional," "too sensitive," "lacking in confidence and work ethic" and "not deserving of respect."

> I was not prejudice when I start working years ago. After years, you see so many things that frustrate you that by *choice* you become prejudice especially, i.e., native people. They treat you as *slave* (white slave).

In the quote above, the white nurse is blaming Native and non-white nurses for "making" her prejudiced. This is a common discourse in North American society, where people of colour are often blamed for bringing racism on themselves by their discrepant behaviour.

> Sometimes the majority of nurses were from another country and would "clump" together and speak in their dialect. (white nurse)

In the above excerpt, it appears that a white nurse is expressing a feeling of being threatened when nurses of colour are interacting on their own terms, whether it is in speaking in their own dialect or being present in larger numbers. In this example, we see the connection between language and the making of people as "other." Would the white nurse feel the same way if a group of nurses were speaking in French or Italian? Or congregating in a large group? As Peggy McIntosh (1990) pointed out, part of enjoying white privilege is to be unaware that most of the time there are white people hanging out together, because it is the norm in our society. Seeing people of colour socializing together challenges that dominant reality, and a few white nurses seem to be troubled by it. In fact, in an earlier chapter, I listed "dispersion" of nurses of colour as a management practice to break non-white nurses' sense of solidarity, security and networking capacity. From a managerial perspective, isolating a nurse reduces her capacity to resist. Underlying this tactic is the sense of feeling threatened by the congregation of a significant number of nurses of colour, animated by stereotypes about their inborn aggression and violence. White nurses who expressed feeling uncomfortable and victimized by nurses of colour speaking their own dialect or socializing together illustrates similar assumptions.

Some white nurses reacted negatively to demands from certain groups, particularly Aboriginal communities, for culturally sensitive healthcare and for self determination of healthcare (Gordon 2004), even though the Canadian government and state policies acknowledge the legitimacy of these demands. A few white nurses perceive them as reverse racism.

Any effort to distribute among or share power with communities of colour is described as being oppressive to white nurses. The following comments are illustrative of this sentiment:

> Statements made about my professional practice were derogatory because I was "Anglo," "you are not one of us, you are not First Nations."

> [I was told] By a person of another profession who indicated that all North American and WASP nurses shouldn't care for persons of colour.... Uncomfortable talking/caring for persons of different race /colours/ethnicity until I know them as there seems to be an automatic assumption that anyone and everyone is looking down on the other.

This last nurse wrote that she resented being labeled a WASP or a European, apparently referring to the racial categories that were provided on the survey form. She insisted that she was Canadian. James (1999: 12) reports that in his classes, it is sometimes typical of British Canadians to describe themselves as "Canadian" and to resist naming their ethnic or racial background. They feel "challenged and uncomfortable." I contend also that in their minds "Canadian" culture is synonymous with British culture, that it is the norm, whereas race and ethnicity are understood to be attributes of "others," those who speak a language other than English and those who are non-white. It betrays a blindness to the privileges one holds as an English-speaking white person in a racist society.

The history of racism in Canada and other settler societies is marked by the imposition of Eurocentric medical models of healthcare, which replaced indigenous or alternative forms of healthcare. This has often resulted in inappropriate diagnosis and treatment of people and has contributed to their poor health. To counter that reality, some communities of colour have organized around demanding the recognition of alternative healthcare, especially forms that are more compatible or sensitive to their own cultures. Perceiving culturally appropriate healthcare or the demand for self determination of healthcare by racialized communities as amounting to reverse racism is similar to equating employment equity programs with reverse racism. Underlying this perception is a resentment towards any proactive programs to address the needs of people of colour, most importantly those arising from their experiences around racism. The reason behind the resentment is an incorrect understanding of what "equality" really entails. A liberal notion of equality implies equal opportunity or access, rather than equality as an end result. Equality of access is seen to be compromised by programs designed to benefit people of colour. They are seen as providing unfair advantages. In recognition of this principle, James (1999: 238) quotes Judge Rosalie Abella:

> Formerly we thought that equity only meant sameness and that treating persons as equals meant treating everyone the same. We now know that treating everyone the same may be to offend the notions of equality....

These "special" programs seem unfair to some whites because they lose their privileged status. For instance, employment equity programs or culturally sensitive healthcare makes it a priority to employ nurses of colour. It must be remembered that such affirmative hiring programs do not mean that white nurses are not being hired. It simply means that previously excluded nurses of colour are now being included in the hiring process and their cross cultural and anti-racist knowledge are being valued as assets, especially in serving patients of colour.

According to Katz et al. (1986), many white Americans feel resentful of Black Americans vis-à-vis such programs as school busing and job quotas. While they support equal opportunity for Blacks, they feel that affirmative action programs provide an unfair advantage to Blacks to the detriment of whites. As discussed in Chapter 2, these theorists further posit that such programs challenge the core American value of individualism, which emphasizes freedom, self reliance, devotion to work and achievement. They see affirmative action programs as "handouts" for which Blacks did not have to work. This clash of core values creates ambivalence in many whites towards Blacks and programs that are created to benefit them by the state. Katz et al. (1986) liken this attitudinal and political ambivalence as a "new" form of racism. The white nurses' comments quoted above may point to a similar viewpoint.

Omi and Winant (1994) comment that affirmative action programs do not constitute "racism in reverse" because they do not essentialize "race," although they racialize people in order to address historical inequalities. The comments from the white nurses quoted above could be re-visited in light of Omi and Winant's assertions. Are the nurses of colour and First Nations nurses that they refer to in their comments essentialist? In other words, are they characterizing whites as being inherently deficient or inferior? The brief comments jotted down by nurses were often not detailed enough to make any conclusions on this question. However, further research could be conducted on these lines. Interestingly, Omi and Winant add that affirmative action programs may affect opportunities for some white people who are not themselves the source of racial injustice and that they should be compensated in some way to avert the charge of "reverse racism."

REVERSE RACISM

A significant number of white nurses who put down comments raised the "reverse racism" argument, i.e., they felt discriminated against by nurses of colour.

> Beginning to feel "reverse" discrimination because I'm Caucasian.

> I experienced reverse racism involving West Indian nurses and so have colleagues in two separate workplaces — not an issue — is the prevailing attitude, but this *DOES exist* and should be addressed.

> I found that racism in the workplace is usually minimal, but it is not something experienced only by non-white people and is equally demoralizing and saddening. In thirty years nursing I only experienced *one* department where it flourished and consequently transferred out of that dept.

Reverse racism implies that persons of colour are discriminating against dominant group members. James (1999: 237) says that the argument of "reverse racism" demonstrates an erroneous understanding of racism. He states that "in so far as racism is supported by a system of inequality and oppression constructed within a society, it is more than individual; it is structural and institutional." Racism requires social power and thus reverse racism is a contradiction in terms. If one is a member of a dominant racial group, other things being equal, that person cannot be put down by a member of the subordinate racial group because the latter does not have the social power to do so. James further clarifies the concept of power as "social" rather than "individual." In other words, racism is not a product of individually powerful white people; rather it is a product of white people as a group being powerful in society and having the ability to influence and make institutional decisions that benefit their group. There is also a historical significance to racism by whites as it represents continuity of a history of white supremacy in many societies

On the other hand, James' preceding conceptualization is based on three erroneous assumptions, i.e., that there are no people of colour in powerful positions in our society, that power only emanates from one's location in the racial hierarchy and that power is either/or, either one has it or not. These assumptions cannot be accepted as a reality in Canada today. As discussed earlier, social power can emanate from a variety of social locations, not only as a result of one's "race," but also because of class, gender, sexuality, age, etc. Hence, it is conceivable that a person in a subordinate racialized social location may enjoy class or gender privilege. So, the more accurate question to pose is: Can a person of colour enjoying some level of social power be racist towards a white person?

What about intra-ethnic power relations? This is an under-researched area of study, but one that has great relevance in a society marked by ethnic diversity. One person of colour could act in a racist manner towards another person of colour who comes from a different ethnic background. There could be a hierarchy of power, so that it is not only whites who have a monopoly over the capacity to be racist.

Negative verbal comments made by nurses or patients of colour that are offensive to white nurses are worth analyzing in light of this discussion.

> I am disappointed/disgusted by this experience [verbal comments from a nurse of colour]. If I, as a white person, said half the comments that I heard I would be facing a disciplinary group. The nurse that offended me was only told about my complaint but not councilled (sic).

> Racial comments were stated about my race from one individual to another, in my presence. I stated I did not appreciate the comments. It went no further. I am simply cautious around anyone and treat all with respect.

Are the two white nurses quoted above victims of racism? We don't have detailed information about the work situations of the nurses who made these comments. But, by and large, we have seen and other authors have written about racism in healthcare settings across the board, where nurses of colour are in subordinate positions. The individual nurses who made put-down remarks towards white nurses are few and far between and do not enjoy any social power as persons of colour. However, they may enjoy social power as managers or supervisors over white nurses and nurses of colour, just as a male doctor of colour would enjoy social class and gender power over nurses in general. If they are indeed in a higher class position within the nursing hierarchy, their class privilege might allow them to make anti-white comments against white nurses working below them. However, this is rare in reality. As we have discussed before, nurses of colour in supervisory positions are often highly monitored, subjected to insubordination by white nurses working below them and held up to standards that are higher than that for white supervisors.

Nurses of colour could be prejudiced because that does not require social power; however, their views are generally not backed up by the policies and procedures of the institution. There is, in other words, no systemic component to their prejudice, i.e., the hospital is not operating with policies, procedures or practices that discriminate against white nurses, nor does the hospital hierarchy reflect a racist division of labour where whites are disadvantaged. The put-down comments are still hurtful, but they are not backed up by hiring, training, promotional and disciplinary policies, procedures and practices. The reason they are not entrenched is that nurses of colour as a group do not have social power within the hospital hierarchy. Rather, it is the other way around. They are in a subordinate position vis-à-vis white nurses and other healthcare workers, both within the hospital and within society at large. My thinking is in line with Omi and Winant (1994: 73), who comment that not all racisms are the same.

SEXISM/CLASSISM SEEN AS REVERSE RACISM

As discussed before, nurses, being predominantly female, are often looked upon as "servants" by men and women in power. Physicians, often male, derive their power from their professional expertise, supported by their lengthy and expensive education and resultant high salaries and prestige. They enjoy a privileged position within healthcare settings. This is reflected in the hierarchies of healthcare institutions (Jacobs 2007). For instance, the Joint Policy and Planning Committee (JPPC), a partnership between the Ontario Hospital Association (OHA) and the Ministry of Health, formed in 1992, which recommends policy directions in healthcare, works closely with the Colleges of Physicians and Surgeons of Ontario and the Ontario Medical Association (OMA), although not so integrally with the Ontario Nurses' Association (ONA) or the College of Nurses of Ontario. Within hospitals, the chief of medical staff is a voting member of the board, while the chief of nursing is not. The following is a comment from a nurse who speaks about a doctor's behaviour towards nurses:

> Bullying, degradation, verbally and emotionally abusive, controlling, manipulative from a black African/Indian physician — he is abusive toward white females, patients as well… Entire staff affected by this dr. This doctor behaved the same way at a previous Ontario hospital and staff were not supported and too intimidated to report resulting in the behaviour repeating itself at another hospital in Ontario. This abuse will probably result in me leaving nursing earlier than previously planned.

Patients are also abusive towards nurses, asserting their power as taxpayers and consumers of medical service. Jacobs (2007) reports that the College of Nurses of Ontario exists to "protect the public interest." In this case "public" represents patients and their families. As such, it has a major disciplinary role on nurses. The following testimonies reveal abusive behaviour towards nurses from patients:

> Men of various colour/ethnicity have made derogatory remarks. It is annoying because I am here to help these people and they do not respect me.

> As different cultures meet, we are more exposed to people who see nurses as personal servants — the level of respect for our profession is lowering as I get older. I do not like my job.

> Some Indian cultures do not respect me because I am female, or make me feel unwelcome because I am white.

Physicians, patients and their family members experience a sense of entitlement to privileges within a healthcare setting. This attitude unfortunately does not escape patients or physicians of colour either. The sexist and classist comments and behaviours that the white nurses talk about are common not only to white female nurses, but to female nurses of colour also. Unfortunately, what is revealed in these comments is that when the harasser is a man of colour and the recipient is a white female, the recipient seems to racialize it only. As a result, harassers of colour are not seen as sexist or classist, but as racist instead. The abusive behaviour of the men is analyzed as emanating from their "backward" and "sexist" cultures rather than from their status as men and as powerful members of a social class. Moreover, these "backward" cultural traits are contrasted to "Canadian culture" (read white, European) as if there is no incidence of sexism and abuse displayed by "Canadian" men. This "us" (meaning white) versus "them" (meaning non-white) sets up a racist discourse, reminiscent of colonial times, when the colonized man was represented always as a brute or despot from whom colonized and white women had to be rescued.

Thus, the despicable sexist and classist abuse that white nurses receive at the hands of doctors and patients of colour is also interpreted in a colonial/racist manner. White nurses subjected to put-downs from physicians and patients of colour interpret these experiences as instances of "reverse racism," which as I have mentioned before negates the destructive nature of racism against people of colour, particularly its systemic and institutionalized forms. How would these same white nurses describe the sexism and classism demonstrated by white doctors and patients? Would their behaviours and comments be attributed to their "race" or ethnic origin? Or, would they be attributed to their individual pathologies, as is so common in the representations of crime where the perpetrator is white as opposed to non-white? How would women of colour describe abusive behaviours of white doctors or of doctors and patients of colour? What makes one set of abusive behaviour racist and sexist, while another set simply sexist? Abusive behaviour towards nurses is clearly sexist when the perpetrators are men and the targets are women. Moreover, the discourse that underlies these abusive and harassing behaviours is that of sexism, i.e., where women are seen as inferior and not deserving of respect and dignity and are expected to withstand these demeaning attitudes towards them. When do such behaviours involve racism in addition to sexism? This occurs when there is a discourse of "race" in addition to one of gender, i.e., when a person is viewed as a member of a racial group with essentialized and inferior characteristics. In order to describe abuse as racist as well as sexist, one has to analyze the interaction between the male and the female in more detail. The quotations provided above do not in all cases provide us with enough background information about the abusive interactions to make any definitive conclusions; however, they are clearly sexist. There is one which is worth a closer look given its overt racialized language:

> Verbally abusive language — "white bitch,""nurses are pigs." Myself and most of my colleagues feel emotionally battered and defenceless when a patient is allowed to be verbally abusive every day of the week. The hospital system seems to be either unwilling or unable to deal with particularly difficult and hostile patients in acute care setting. Please note this patient is not confused or being treated for a psychiatric disorder.

A non-white patient characterizing a woman nurse as a "white bitch" is definitely an indication of racialization in addition to sexualization. This comment is racist as a speech act, in addition to being clearly sexist in my view. The patient is using his social power as a man and as someone being served to put-down a woman who has a lower social standing in terms of gender, particularly one who is "serving," although she has more social power on the "race" front. The patient takes advantage of his current position of being served to note that the nurse is white and uses that detail to put her down as a woman. I would hasten to add though that his racism is different from the racism of a white patient or doctor in the same setting because of the institutional structure, which supports racism against non-whites. The racism displayed by the patient in the quotation above is an instance of individual racism, In this case racism directed at a white woman. Is this anti-white racism backed up by institutional power? I would say not.

What is significant about abuse perpetrated by patients as described by white nurses (and nurses of colour) is that hospital management and existing policies do not seem to be able to do anything to deter this kind of behaviour as a rule. Doctors, patients and their family members are able to continue with their abuse of nurses as the following comments illustrate:

> I feel management at any level of the hospital should not allow pts. (clients) to refuse a nurse's care because of sex, race, colour, ethnicity. I'm tired of men from countries when women are nothing been allow to refuse a female nurse's care, because it is not allow in his country. *This is Canada.*

It appears, therefore, that given this institutional context the individual racism and sexism of some doctors and patients of colour against white nurses is allowed to continue without much deterrence. However, it is allowed to continue not because of systemic racism against whites but rather because hospital and other healthcare settings are so entrenched in classism, sexism and a corporate culture of consumerism. The latter elements allow male doctors and patients to practise racism in addition to sexism and classism. Unfortunately, as discussed before, the white nurse who is the victim of such behaviours also has a racialized response because she describes her oppressor's actions as emanating from his "race" and fails to see how his sex/gender and status play major roles in the continuation of his behaviour. Moreover, he is identified as a non-Canadian, as someone outside the nation, in contrast with her, a "true" Canadian, who is more advanced and civilized.

Jacobs (2007) argues that "nursing is a dangerous profession and there are occupational health and safety implications," with verbal, physical and emotional violence being common. She considers abuse in hospital settings to be a culmination of many systemic and interpersonal factors. In fact, nurses often suffer physical assaults. Jacobs notes that such treatment of nurses has been analyzed as an example of violence against women in our society. It is important to emphasize that the abuse generally emanates from patriarchy rather than "race" or "ethnicity," although racialization processes can complicate this analysis, as in examples discussed above. Varied, new and intersecting forms of racism, sexism and classism have arisen as a result of changing social relations.

What is significant in the case of violence against nurses is the inaction by employing and affiliated institutions. For example, Jacobs (2007) discusses the fact that until 2004, the College of Nurses produced materials on client/patient abuse but not on the abuse of nurses. The view that "patients are always right" or "physicians are untouchable" can perpetuate systemic sexism, classism and racism against nurses. The same institution that does not react to racial harassment from white physicians and patients also does not react to sexist or classist harassment from white and non-white physicians and patients. Other forms of discriminatory behaviour towards nurses, e.g., ableism, are also allowed to continue in this environment.

"PLAYING THE RACE CARD" TO HIDE INCOMPETENCE

Discourses of "incompetence" and "playing the race card" are evident in white nurses' comments. According to them, many nurses of colour are incompetent and are trying to defend themselves by claiming to be victims of discrimination.

> I have clients requesting not a certain ethnicity of personal support worker. I tell them I am booking for the role, not the individual. Everyone is judge-

mental against someone. Being in the majority does not negate reverse discrimination, e.g., covering for inadequacy by blaming others for judging on race when it's really a skill (or lack of) issue. I believe racism still exists, but I've been fortunate to not be negatively impacted thus far.

I feel every nurse is a human being deserving of RESPECT! It doesn't matter what color, race or ethnicity you are. I treat everyone equal. It really bothers me that *some* Black nurses scream discrimination when you approach them with an issue as far as their performance. Their first response is "you are harassing me because I'm black!" When will this stop?

One of the things that is evident in these quotes is that the white nurses have some ambivalence in how they understand and handle racism. On the positive side, the first nurse says, "I am booking for the role, not the individual," which means that she does not cater to specific demands of racist patients. The second nurse similarly says, "I feel every nurse is a human being… I treat everyone equal." However, they also refer to the nurse of colour "playing the race card" to deny her own incompetence, and they label this denial and the counter charge of racism as "reverse racism." The following excerpts also point to this sort of labelling.

I find that "reverse racism" is apparent — we are not "permitted" (by this I mean we let it go to avoid further problems) to report fellow staff who leave work undone or sit and chat instead of working for fear they will claim it's because I'm black, Indian, Asian, etc.

There are clearcut incidences of "reverse" racism in the workplace. This nurse has used it for years to cover her abrasive nurse-patient style and job performance issues, i.e., if she is criticized in *any* way it's all due to "RACISM."

Since these white nurses have had trouble being affirmed in their criticisms of non-white nurses, they perceive themselves as "victims" of their non-white colleagues and of anti-racism and human rights policies. As stated earlier, such perceptions reveal a lack of understanding of the systemic power that underpins racialized relationships. The existence of human rights and anti-racism policies may have reversed the power balance within institutions to make it more difficult to label nurses of colour as incompetent. These white nurses perceive a limitation in their power to criticize their colleagues of colour and they apparently resent this new reality. At the same time, they vehemently insist that they believe in equality and that everyone is deserving of respect. We see here a juxtaposition of democratic ideals and racist practice. There is a denial of the historical reality of racism against people of colour in these quotes, rather than an acknowledgement of the defensive action of nurses of colour against the charge of incompetence, and the subsequent charge of racism against their white accusers is viewed as "reverse racism." Carl James[2] clarifies the phrase "reverse racism" as a misnomer. It is either racism or it is not racism. As discussed earlier in this chapter and in Chapter 2, it is possible for people of colour in powerful positions to exercise individual racism, but not systemic or institutional racism. Be that as it may, is the denial of the charge of incompetence and the counter charge of racism against a white accuser a sign of racism? I maintain not. It is a racialized response given a history of institutionalized racism against nurses of colour; however, the reaction of the nurse of colour is not essentializing the white nurse or her behaviour on the basis of her whiteness.

> I am white — reported the flagrantly poor care of a nurse who is black. The nurse threatened to complain to HRC. The nurse mentioned had provided sub-standard patient care i.e., documentation poor, care of an incapable of self care patient — unhygienic, irregular vital signs — ignored! Miscarried fetus was left in a towel in the room bereaved mother was staying in. I was threatened with Human Rights Commission reporting as "I criticized her because she is black" in her view. As a social democratic person who is not racist this was very disturbing to me. I was laid off from that job in __ and left demoralized because of this.

It is not clear in this quote whether the white nurse was laid off as a result of her accusation of the Black nurse or as a result of a general downsizing exercise. However, as in earlier excerpts, the white nurse was accused of being racist as a result of her criticism of the Black nurse's practice.

In critiquing these white nurses' comments, I am not saying that nurses of colour do not make mistakes or that they are never incompetent. Rather, I am cautioning against judging the alleged incompetence as emanating from her "race" or the denial of incompetence as "playing the race card." "Race cards" may be played by all parties. In a racially charged workplace culture, wrongful accusations of incompetence have been rampant against nurses of colour. My research shows that nurses of colour are often held up to higher standards as far as competence is concerned. For instance, while white nurses may be routinely making errors in documentation, nurses of colour are being formally charged and disciplined for not documenting and charting properly. In other words, policies and procedures are being rigorously followed in the case of nurses of colour but not so in the case of white nurses. There is differential treatment where performance evaluations and discipline are concerned.

There have also been cases where nurses of colour were set up to be incompetent through excessive monitoring or scapegoating, as in Evelyn's case in Chapter 4. Her ability to perform effectively as a nurse was affected because of harassment. She was accused and disciplined for alleged incompetence, while other professionals on the scene were untouched. Standards of competence must be consistent in application irrespective of the "race" or ethnicity of the nurse. If a nurse of colour is found to be incompetent according to such standards, she should be subjected to the same processes that white nurses are subjected to, including provision of re-training, progressive discipline, etc. Moreover, if she is alleged to be incompetent, there should be an examination of whether harassment was implicated at any stage and how that can be addressed. Further, institutions need to monitor whether there are patterns of incompetence being identified with nurses of colour. In other words, if nurses of colour are over-represented among those marked as "incompetent," then management (in conjunction with the relevant unions) needs to review performance appraisals, training and disciplinary measures to analyze whether these are contributing to systemic racism.

The discourses revealed through the nurses' comments show the complexity of how racism operates, particularly in its interlocking nature, and how difficult it is to dismantle. Educators have to begin from received ideological positions and unravel the discriminatory discourses that underlie them. The process promises to be extremely challenging.

NOTES

1. I am grateful for feedback received from Dr. Carl James on this chapter. Some of the analysis here emerged out of a dialogue with him.
2. Personal communication.

7. THE WAY AHEAD

In this study, I set out to explore the dynamics of systemic racism in nursing as it manifests itself in Ontario. I began with a simple notion of systemic racism as arising from conscious or unconscious policies, procedures and practices that adversely affect people of colour. I argued that in order to understand systemic racism, one also has to understand other forms of racism connected with it. Moreover, racism exists in interlocking relationships with other discourses such as sexism, classism and able-ism.

Four forms of racism were discussed, including everyday racism based on individual behaviour, systemic racism, common-sensical beliefs and racist/colonialist discourses. I described these forms as being on a continuum. One can also describe racism as being cyclical, one form resting on the other, so that the manifestation of one form usually ensures the existence of the other forms, even though they may not be immediately visible.

Individual behavioural racism or everyday racism is the form most frequently identified by nurses of colour in conversations, interviews and grievances. However, the connections between this form and the more hidden systemic and discursive forms need complex, multi-layered analyses, where the institution's employment systems and workforce are studied. Such analyses require case studies of particular workplaces. In this regard, my earlier study of Northwestern General Hospital (NWGH) is referred to in this report.

A survey that I conducted with ONA members revealed that most nurses of colour have experienced everyday forms of racism, including being infantilized and marginalized. Most reported being "put down," insulted or degraded because of race/ethnicity/colour. A significant proportion of nurses, non-white and white, report having witnessed an incident where a nurse was treated differently because of his/her race/ethnicity/colour. The person subjected to racism is almost always a nurse of colour while the perpetrator is typically white.

The largest proportion of "putdowners" were colleagues, followed by patients, doctors, managers and others. This has implications for the ONA and other unions, as well as for employers who are interested in instituting anti-racist harassment policies. For instance, effective co-worker harassment policies are necessary to address harassment by colleagues. Educational programs around race and racism are essential to further an understanding. Effective policies around harassment from patients are also necessary. Institutions also need to initiate consciousness-raising, education and training to facilitate the utilization of such policies, which need to be monitored and evaluated so that they can be made more effective over time.

Nurses subjected to racial harassment and to racism in general need to be supported by institutions. Currently, this is not always happening, and whatever support nurses receive is through their own community organizations, families and friends. Institutionally speaking, their experiences are often denied. Nurses subjected to everyday racism report being affected emotionally, physically, mentally and in other ways. Many are quitting their job, taking early retirement or leaving the profession because of the lack of support. Those who remain suffer the consequences of working in a poisoned environment, often sustaining long-term ill health.

An examination of racism in healthcare settings provides us with a window on how it is dealt with personally and systemically in an environment marked by vulnerability, a result of the seriousness of illness and the prospect of life and death. Vulnerability also results from the rigid hierarchies that characterize healthcare institutions and nurses' location within these structures as women and as racialized workers.

Many nurses subjected to racial incidents do not take any action because of fear, socialization, lack of progress from previous actions and lack of understanding of racism. Most nurses who take action use personal assertiveness, talking to their supervisor, talking to the ONA, filing incident reports and filing grievances. However, only a few nurses filed grievances, and most of those were dismissed due to lack of evidence. This is of concern since it deters nurses from using the grievance procedure to address racial harassment. This might also alienate nurses of colour from the organized labour movement. In comparison, personal strategies to fight harassment are often more effective. However, these are not effective against more systemic and complex harassment.

Systemic racism in nursing is suggested by a number of factors. Although recent statistical breakdowns of the nursing workforce by racial background in Ontario were not available, there are indications that racial segregation still exists in most hospitals. Nurses of colour are often segregated to the lower levels of nursing, which require less education, skill and competency in comparison to middle and higher levels. Nurses of colour are also segregated to less desirable areas of work, often characterized by lack of advancement. More nurses of colour compared to white nurses report that their race/ethnicity/colour influence where they work.

Employment equity in nursing on the basis of race should be a top priority for all healthcare institutions. Despite the problematic nature of racial categorization discussed in Chapter 2, there is a dire need for the collection of "race" data so that patterns of segregation can be better studied and addressed. Employment equity should be proactive, should include educational programs for all levels of nurses and administrators and should establish goals and timetables. Employment equity should not be limited to lower level positions, but should also address middle and upper levels, including supervisory/

managerial positions. The indepth interviews with senior nurses of colour revealed that the "glass ceiling" is very much a reality for them.

Racial segregation occurs systemically, i.e., through policies, procedures and practices within the employment systems, and employment equity programs need to address these systemic barriers. More nurses of colour compared to white nurses reported that their hirings, promotions, access to training, accommodation due to disability, sick leave provisions, performance reviews and disciplinary actions were affected by their race/ethnicity/colour. This is a very significant finding of this study and has policy implications.

Nurses of colour mentioned lack of mentoring, lack of information, "lack of fit" and being by-passed as ways in which their promotional chances are lowered. More nurses of colour, including a majority of Black/African Canadian nurses, compared to white nurses, reported that their relationships with their managers are affected by their race/ethnicity/colour. Presumably, these negative relationships adversely affect their chances for promotion.

Pursuing higher education is how many nurses of colour try to compensate for barriers to promotions, even though they often experience racism within nursing training institutions as well. Although this was not a focus of my research, many nurses talked about these experiences. University and community college programs need to be examined to remove systemic barriers for nursing students of colour to promote educational equity. This is a pre-requisite for promoting employment equity.

Although my survey did not yield a great deal of information regarding foreign credential recognition, a number of ONA grievances and arbitration decisions, as well as the case study of the de-registration and subsequent unemployment of foreign trained nurses in 1994, reveal that this is an area for future research. With the requirement of a BScN for all new nurses, there are concerns among anti-racism advocates as to its effects on new registered nurse immigrants coming from outside Canada. How will their credentials be recognized? Will they be facilitated into getting their Canadian registration as nurses or will they be streamed into lower levels of nursing? Given the nursing shortage, the latter would be unfortunate both for the immigrant nurses as well as for Canadian consumers. At the time of writing, the Ministry of Training, Colleges and Universities had funded a bridge training program called Creating Access to Regulated Employment (CARE) for Nurses (http://care4nurses.org) to provide supports and services to internationally educated nurses living in Ontario to facilitate their transition into their profession. It is important to monitor how the participants in CARE fare in the process of finding a nursing job, whether it is full-time or part-time, level of skills, salary and so on.

An area that could be further explored is the lack of accommodation due to disability for nurses of colour. The survey did not reveal much data in this area, but some interviews with and grievances filed by disabled nurses of colour indicate that further research is required.

There is also merit in research being conducted for particular ethnic/ racial groups as my survey results indicate that there are differences among different groups, even in their experience of racism. Each non-white community has had a different historical relationship to white/European peoples. Therefore, each group may be subjected to different sets of racist discourses, which give rise to different racialized relationships. Research should be initiated on the particular experiences of Aboriginal nurses. Only one Aboriginal nurse responded to my survey, and I did not report on her answers to maintain confidentiality and anonymity. My survey indicates that anti-Black racism is prevalent in nursing. In almost every category, Black/African nurses reported that race/ethnicity/colour influenced their employment experience.

The labour market for nurses in Canada fluctuates. The number of registered nurses in full-time nursing increased from 41,064 in 1999 to 43, 899 in 2000, while part-timers went down over the same period (CIHI 2000). Employment in hospitals as well as in community health centres went up dramatically during this time. However, the number of nurses employed in nursing in Ontario per 10,000 population had declined since 1995 from 72 to 69.7 (Samuelson 2002). In the 1990s, many disillusioned nurses left the province or the country. Thousands of Canadian nurses have been moving to the U.S. for full-time jobs since in 1990s (Taylor 2008). Hagey, Choudhry et al (2001) write that immigrant nurses are being sought to fill the void, but under what conditions?

Letters from ONA members in *ONA Vision* as well as letters in national newspapers (Zeltric 2002) indicate that nurses are overworked due to the nursing shortage. Many work without break times and on overtime hours. "They are among the sickest workers in Ontario" (Samuelson 2002; *ONA Vision* 2005). Many nurses still feel a lack of respect for their profession demonstrated by the lack of administrative consultation with them. These are less than ideal conditions for positive working relationships to develop among healthcare professionals. These conditions are a disincentive for young women and men to consider nursing as a career.

In 2003, the Registered Nurses Association on Ontario (RNAO) estimated that 43 percent of nurses worked on a part-time or casual basis (Urquhart 2003), while most of these nurses would prefer to work full-time in nursing. Apart from the existing working conditions making nurses sicker, it appeared that nurses working two or more part-time jobs in different hospitals have contributed to spreading deadly diseases like SARS and West Nile, which compromised the health of patients and nurses. The Registered Nurses Association of Ontario continues to call for boosting the full-time employment in nursing (*Toronto Star* 2003) in order to provide good patient care and safer workloads for nurses. They estimate that about 15,000 more nursing positions would be needed to return to an acceptable population-nurse ratio.

The Liberal government in Ontario has promised to hire 9,000 nurses by 2011 and has created a program to guarantee seven and a half months of full-time work to new graduates (Taylor 2008). At the same time, the short-age of full-time jobs in Canada motivates many young nurses to seek jobs in the U.S. A new crisis is around the corner with over 40 percent of Canada's nurses being eligible to retire in the next five years (Ogilvie 2008).

One would like to think that racism in nursing would be less of a concern in a labour market where demand's up relative to the supply of registered nurses. However, the problem of morale for nurses evident in the 1980s and 1990s appears to be just as prevalent today. It is clear that healthcare is in a worse crisis today than it was in 2003, when new resources were called for to "reform and renew" the healthcare system (Romanow 2003). Neo-liberal policies of privatization and downloading continue to be strengthened in different ways. De-institutionalization results in funding being diverted into cheaper community-based care, including community clinics, home care and nursing care, heavily dependent on lower paid workers, workers of colour and unpaid female workers in households. A Supreme Court ruling voted 4–3 in favour of a Quebec man (awaiting hip surgery) who challenged provincial law that prevents individuals from buying health insurance for private services already provided by public healthcare (Gordon and Mills 2005).

Historically, the relationship between unions and racism has been prob-lematic, a topic I have explored elsewhere (Das Gupta 2007, 1998). In this study, I have not discussed the role of the union, the ONA, in tackling racism in nursing. This was necessary in order to limit the research parameters as the study's primary focus was on racism in healthcare settings. However, a focus on the ONA in terms of how it has handled racism among its members would be a worthwhile undertaking. The ONA's capacity to advocate for its members of colour in the area of racial harassment would be greatly enhanced if rac-ism was a priority area for it and if the ONA consciously addressed racism within its own structures, policies and practices. There are some suggestions that the latter has not happened yet.

As mentioned at the outset, the recommendation to conduct the research came out of the ONA's Racially Diverse Caucus in 2000. Since this study was conducted using a collaborative research process with the ONA, I was in close consultation with the ONA's Equity Specialist throughout the research and writing process. The final report was delivered in March 2003. The enthusiasm and interest the ONA expressed at the outset of the research was not evident once the report had been produced. About a year passed during which time I did not get any feedback from the ONA. Upon enquiring as to the status of the report, I was told that the report had been announced in

Vision (2003), a magazine for ONA members, in which it was indicated that the executive summary was available to members. The full report was given to the board of directors, and local executives and human rights and equity representatives were informed that they could obtain the full report upon request. The Human Rights and Equity Team of the ONA was asked to make recommendations on how the report could be best utilized by membership and staff. One of the team's recommendations was to present the report to local executive members to assist them in addressing local issues.

Soon after, I was invited to present the highlights of the report to a meeting of ONA area coordinators in March 2004. The presentation was followed by a question and answer period. Some local leaders noted that the report had been very useful to them in understanding their situation. A handful of vocal nurses of colour challenged the ONA leadership, saying that the report had not been made accessible to members. They called for the report to be mailed out to all local leaders, rather than leaving the onus on them to obtain a copy.

In 2005, the report became the basis of a presentation made by the ONA to the OHRC on racism and racial discrimination. I was also informed that the president and chief executive officer of the ONA were presenting a summary of the report and its implications for the union at the International Council of Nurses in Taipei (Haslam-Stroud and Bell 2005). That paper delineated the ONA's educational activities emanating from my study. Apparently, the ONA has incorporated parts of the report, particularly personal testimonies, into its human rights and equity workshops for members. It is also mentioned that the ONA's board members had completed diversity training, although no details were provided as to its characteristics, length, effectiveness and follow-up. It was mentioned that similar training will be extended to staff members as well. Beyond the union, the ONA made recommendations to the Ontario Hospital Association, the employer organization representing 159 public hospitals, to develop joint educational programs for hospital staff. The ONA has also had discussions with the College of Nurses of Ontario and the registered Nurses Association of Ontario with regard to co-worker racism. Whether these ideas and initiatives will be followed up and implemented remains to be seen. The experience in other unions reminds us that success in implementing anti-racism policies depends on the activism of members of colour and other anti-racist supporters inside and outside the union. Policies and research reports do not necessarily mean that racism has been tackled and controlled. As argued in this study, racism can co-exist within institutions with glossy anti-racist and human rights laws, policies, staff members and elected officials. Change is brought about not through institutionalizing anti-racism or equity, but through making structural changes that allow the voices of members of colour to be heard in a meaningful way, not as tokenistic gestures.

Certainly, collective agreements and grievance and arbitration procedures can be powerful mechanisms in redressing racial harassment. Unfortunately, these mechanisms do not work in favour of workers of colour if the will to deploy these mechanisms to affect change is not readily there. For example, Calliste (1996: 381) reminds us that when the nurses of NWGH came out with their complaints of racial harassment against their employer, the ONA did not show a willingness to support the complainants until the Coalition for Black Nurses, initiated by the Congress of Black Women of Canada, lobbied them to do so. Nurses and Friends Against Discrimination (NAFAD), formed around the same time, also challenged the ONA to stop collaborating with employers during grievances and to stop pressurizing members to settle grievances in return for withdrawal of human rights complaints or imposition of gag orders. Unions themselves need anti-racist policies, procedures and practices so that they can be equipped to deal with racism as it affects their members in their workplaces and within the union. As my study indicates, co-worker harassment is a serious problem that needs to be addressed. Changing the representation of the union is a crucial first step in initiating an anti-racist change process, so that it is not perceived as a white union, but as a diverse organization accountable to all its members in all their diversity.

The other roadblock to fighting racism through grievances and arbitration hearings is that nurses often face reprisals for complaining against their employers. Hagey et al. (2001) interviewed nine immigrant nurses of colour who had filed grievances through the ONA. The nurses reported being isolated and subjected to punishment from employers and colleagues. They also experienced physical stress, emotional pain and loss of material comforts, e.g., losing their house or car as a result of their grievances. Moreover, their findings suggest that some nurses perceived the ONA as siding with management in their grievances. In fact, the nurses' grievance and arbitration processes were such negative experiences that the authors of the study argued for exploring alternative justice models, particularly ones that do not rely on an adversarial approach.

Racism is a complex problem and we need a multi-pronged strategy to address it. A diversity of methods is required, including worker support, educational efforts, community coalitions, union grievance procedures, human rights commissions, equity legislation and the courts. While we have some of these mechanisms in place, they are not always effective. Anti-racist agents have to be constantly vigilant and make institutions and bodies accountable to community groups, particularly those of colour.

REFERENCES

Armstrong, Pat, Carol Amaratunga, Jocelyn Bernier, Karen Grant, Ann Pederson and Kay Wilson. 2001. *Exposing Privatization: Women and Healthcare Reform in Canada.* Aurora: Garamond Press.

Armstrong, Pat, and Hugh Armstrong. 1990. *Theorizing Women's Work.* Toronto: Garamond Press.

_____. 1996. *Wasting Away: The Undermining of Canadian Healthcare.* Toronto: University of Toronto Press.

Bannerji, Himani. 1995. *Thinking Through: Essays on Feminism, Marxism and Anti-Racism.* Toronto: Women's Press.

Banton, Michael. 1987. "The Classification of Races in Europe and North America: 1700–1850." *International Social Science Journal* 39(1): 32–46.

Benjamin, Lorna Akua. 2003. *The Black/Jamaican Criminal: The Making of Ideology.* PhD thesis, University of Toronto.

Billig, Michael et al. 1998. *Ideological Dilemmas: A Social Psychology of Everyday Thinking.* London: Sage Publications.

Bottomore, Tom (ed.). 1983. *A Dictionary of Marxist Thought.* Cambridge, MA: Harvard University Press.

Brand, Dionne. 1987. "Black Women and Work: The Impact of Racially Constructed Gender Roles on the Sexual Division of Labour: Part 1." *Fireweed* 25: 28–37.

_____. 1999. "Black Women and Work: The Impact of Racially Impacted Gender Roles on the Sexual Division of Labour." In Enakshi Dua and Angela Robertson (eds.), *Scratching the Surface: Canadian Anti-Racist Feminist Thought.* Toronto: Women's Press.

Broad, D. 2000. *Hollow Work, Hollow Society? Globalization and the Casual Labour Problem in Canada.* Halifax: Fernwood.

Caissey, Ina. 1994. "Discrimination and Racism in Ontario's Healthcare Industry." Presentation to the City of North York's Community, Race and Ethnic Relations Committee, Ontario Nurses' Association (ONA). October 13.

Calliste, Agnes. 1993. "Women of 'Exceptional Merit': Immigration of Caribbean Nurses to Canada." *Canadian Journal of Women and the Law* 6: 85–102.

_____. 1996. "Anti-Racism Organizing and Resistance in Nursing: African Canadian Women." *Canadian Review of Sociology and Anthropology* 33 (3): 361–90.

Calliste, Agnes, and George J. Sefa Dei (eds.). 2000. *Anti-Racist Feminism: Critical Race and Gender Studies.* Halifax, NS: Fernwood Publishing.

Campbell, Marie. 1988. "Management as 'Ruling': A Class Phenomenon in Nursing." *Studies in Political Economy* 27, Autumn.

Campbell, Marie, and Ann Manicom (eds.). 1995. *Knowledge, Experience and Ruling Relations: Studies in the Social Organization of Knowledge.* Toronto: University of Toronto Press.

Campbell, Marie. 1988. "Management as 'Ruling': A Class Phenomenon in Nursing." *Studies in Political Economy* 27, Autumn.

Canadian Nurses Association and the Canadian Hospital Association. 1990. *Nurse Retention and Quality of Work Life: A National Perspective.* Ottawa.

Carlisle, Daloni. 1990. "Trying to Open Door." *Nursing Times* 86, 18 (May 2).

Castagna, Maria, and George J. Sefa Dei. 2000. "An Historical Overview of the Application of the Race Concept in Social Practice." In Agnes Calliste and George J. Sefa Dei (eds.), *Anti-Racist Feminism*. Halifax, NS: Fernwood Publishing.

Cernetig, Miro. 2005. "Looking Over Their Shoulders." *Toronto Star*. Sunday, February 13: A8.

CIHI (Canadian Institute for Health Information). 2000. "Supply and Distribution of Registered Nurses in Canada 2000." Available at <http://secure.cihi.ca/cihiweb/dispPage.jsp?cw_page=AR_20_E > accessed October 2008.

Clement, Wallace, and Leah F. Vosko (eds.). 2003. *Changing Canada: Political Economy as Transformation*. Montreal: McGill-Queen's University Press.

Collins, Enid, et al. 1997. "Research Toward Equity in the Professional Life of Immigrants: A Study of Nursing in the Metropolis." Available at <http://ceris.metropolis.net/Virtual%20Library/RFPReports/Collins1997.pdf> accessed October 2008.

Commission on Systemic Racism on the Ontario Criminal Justice System. 1994. *Racism Behind Bars: The Treatment of Blacks and Other Racial Minority Prisoners in Ontario Prisons*. Toronto: Queen's Printer for Ontario.

Connelly, M. Patricia, and Pat Armstrong (eds.). 1992. *Feminism in Action: Studies in Political Economy*. Toronto: Canadian Scholars' Press.

Court of Appeal for Ontario. 1992. *Between Her Majesty the Queen and Carlton Parks*. October 20.

Cranford, Cynthia J., and Leah F. Vosko. 2006. "Conceptualizing Precarious Employment." In Leah F. Vosko (ed.), *Precarious Employment: Understanding Labour Market Insecurity in Canada*. Montreal: McGill-Queen's University Press.

Das Gupta, Tania. 1994. "Analytical Report on the Human Rights Case Involving Northwestern General Hospital." Toronto, March 28.

_____. 1996a. *Racism and Paid Work*. Toronto: Garamond Press, 1996.

_____. 1996b. "Anti-Black Racism in Nursing in Ontario." *Studies in Political Economy* 51 (Fall): 97–116.

_____. 1998. "Anti-Racism and the Organized Labour Movement." In Vic Satzewich (ed.), *Racism and Social Inequality in Canada*. Toronto: Thompson Educational Publishing.

_____. 2000. "Families of Native Peoples, Immigrants and People of Colour." In Nancy Mandell and Ann Duffy (eds.), *Canadian Families: Diversity, Conflict & Change* Toronto: Harcourt Brace.

_____. 2003. "Understanding Racial Discrimination." Paper presented at the Second Annual Human Rights Symposium: Focus on Racial Discrimination, Osgoode Hall Law School of York University, Toronto, May 22.

_____. 2007. "Racism and the Labour Movement." In Gerald Hunt and David Rayside (eds.), *Equalizing Labour: Union Responses to Equity in Canada*. Toronto, University of Toronto Press.

Davis, Angela. 1981. *Women, Race and Class*. London: Women's Press.

de Wolff. 2000. *Breaking the Myth of Flexible Work: Contingent Work in Toronto*. Toronto: Contingent Workers Project.

Dei, George J. Sefa. 1998. "The Politics of Educational Change: Taking Anti-Racism Education Seriously." In Vic Satzewich (ed.), *Racism and Social Inequality in Canada*. Toronto: Thompson Educational Pub.

Delgado, Richard, and Jean Stefancic (eds.). 2000. *Critical Race Theory: The Cutting Edge.* Philadelphia: Temple University Press.

Depradine, Lincoln. 1994. "Call For Probe of Hospital Racism." *Share* 17 (32): 2. Dec. 1.

_____. 1995. "CBWC·Hopes to Aid Nurses." *Share* 17 (45): 2. March 2.

_____. 1995a. "Branson Hospital Pays Up." *Share* 18 (38): 1. Jan. 4.

_____. 1995b. "Nurse Angry Over Delay." *Share* 18 (38): 1. Jan. 4.

Devlin, Richard F. n.d. "Comments: We Can't Go On Together with Suspicious Minds: Judicial Bias and Racialized Perspective in R. v. R.D.S." *Dalhousie Law Journal* 18: 408–46.

Donkoh, Sam. 1997. "Rights Body Failing Workers." *Share* 20 (11): 1.

Doris Marshall Institute (DMI), and Arnold Minors. 1994. *Ethno-Racial Equality: A Distant Goal? An Interim Report to Northwestern General Hospital.* Toronto.

Dovidioi, John F., and Samuel L. Gaertner (eds.). 1986. *Prejudice, Discrimination and Racism.* Orlando: Academic Press.

Dua, Enakshi. 1999. "Beyond Diversity: Exploring the Ways in Which the Discourse of Race Has Shaped the Institution of the Nuclear Family." In Enakshi Dua and Angela Robertson (eds.), *Scratching the Surface: Canadian Anti-Racist Feminist Thought.* Toronto: Women's Press.

Dua, Enakshi, and Angela Robertson. 1999. *Scratching the Surface: Canadian Anti-Racist Feminist Thought.* Toronto: Women's Press.

Edmonds, Susan. 2001. "Racism as a Determinant of Women's Health: A Workshop." Toronto: York University, September 17.

Essed, Philomena. 1991. *Understanding Everyday Racism: An Interdisciplinary Theory.* Newbury Park: Sage Publications.

Fanfair, Ron. 1994. "OHRC 'Bungling' Nurses' Cases." *Share* 17, 34 (Dec 15): 3.

Feagin, Joe R. 2003. "Death By Discrimination." Available at <diversityhealthnetwork@yahoogroups.com?> accessed January 15, 2003.

Frontlines. 2005. ONA Spring.

Galabuzi, Grace-Edward. 2006. *Canada's Economic Apartheid: The Social Exclusion of Racialized Groups in the New Century.* Toronto: Canadian Scholars' Press.

Gilroy, Paul. 2000. *Against Race: Imagining Political Culture Beyond the Color Line.* Cambridge: Belknap Press of Harvard University Press.

Gordon, Mary. 2004. "Aboriginal Concerns to Get $700M Increase." *Toronto Star*, Sept 14: A8.

Gordon, Sean, and Mills, Andrew. 2005. "Timely Healthcare a Basic Right, Supreme Court Says." *Toronto Star* June 10: A1.

Gray, Stan. 1994. "Hospitals and Human Rights." *Our Times* 13 (6): 17–20.

Grinspun, Doris. 2000. "Taking Care of the Bottom Line: Shifting Paradigms in Hospital Management." In Diana L. Gustafson (ed.), *Care and Consequences: The Impact of Healthcare Reform.* Halifax, NS: Fernwood.

Gustafson, Diana L. 2002. *Cultural Sensitivity as a Problematic in Ontario Nursing Policy and Education: An Integrated Feminist Contextual Analysis.* Phd thesis, University of Toronto.

Hagey, Rebecca, Ushi Choudhry, Sepali Guruge, Jane Turrittin, Enid Collins, Ruth Lee. 2001. "Immigrant Nurses' Experience of Racism." *Journal of Nursing Scholarship* 33, 4 (December).

Hagey, Rebecca, Lillie Lum, Robert MacKay, Jane Turritin and Evelyn Brody. 2001. "Exploring Transformative Justice in the Employment of Nurses: Toward Reconstructing Race Relations and the Dispute Process." Unpublished report to the Law Commission of Canada, November.

Hamilton, Roberta. 1996. *Gendering the Vertical Mosaic: Feminist Perspectives on Canadian Society.* Toronto: Copp Clarke Ltd.

Haslam-Stroud, Linda, and Lesley Bell. 2005. "Racism in Nursing." Paper presented at International Council of Nurses (ICN) 23rd Quadrennial Congress, Taipei.

Head, Wilson. 1985. *An Exploratory Study of Attitudes and Perceptions of Minority and Majority Group Healthcare Workers.* Ontario: Ontario Human Rights Commission.

Henry, Frances, and Carol Tator, Winston Mattis, and Tim Rose. 2000. *The Colour of Democracy: Racism in Canadian Society.* Toronto: Harcourt Brace.

Hill-Collins, Patricia. 1990. *Black Feminist Thought: Knowledge, Consciousness and the Politics of Empowerment.* New York: Routledge.

Hine, Darlene Clark. 1989. *Black Women in White.* Bloomington: Indiana University Press.

hooks, bell. 1981. *Ain't I A Woman: Black Women and Feminism.* Boston: Southend Press.

_____. 1992. *Black Looks: Race and Representation.* Toronto: Between the Lines.

Hum, Derek, and Wayne Simpson. 2007. "Revisiting Equity and Labour: Immigration, Gender, Minority Status, and Income Differentials in Canada." *Race and Racism in 21st Century Canada.* Toronto: Broadview Press.

Institute of Race Relations. 1982. *Patterns of Racism Book 2.* England: Institute of Race Relations.

Jacobs, Merle. 2007. *The Cappucino Principle: Health, Culture and Social Justice in the Workplace.* Toronto: de Sitter Publications.

Jakubowski, Lisa Marie. 1997. *Immigration and the Legalization of Racism.* Halifax, NS: Fernwood Publishing.

James, Carl E. 1999. *Seeing Ourselves: Exploring Race, Ethnicity and Culture.* Toronto: Thompson Educational Publishing.

Katz, Irwin, Joyce Wackenhut and R. Glen Hass. 1986. "Racial Ambivalence, Value Duality and Behavior." In John F. Dovidio and Samuel L. Gaertner (eds.), *Prejudice, Discrimination and Racism.* Orlando: Academic Press.

Keung, Nicholas, and Christopher Hutsul. 2003. "What Racial Profiling Feels Like." *Toronto Star,* Tuesday, April 1: B2.

Khayatt, Didi. 1994. "The Boundaries of Identity at the Intersections of Race, Class, Gender." *Canadian Woman Studies* 14(2): 6–12.

Kirchheimer, Sid. 2003. "Racism Should be a Public Health Issue." Available at <http://www.medscape.com/viewarticle/447757> accessed October 2008.

Kirkham, Della. 1998. "The Reform Party of Canada: A Discourse on Race, Ethnicity and Equality." In Vic Stazewich (ed.), *Racism and Social Inequality in Canada.* Toronto: Thompson.

Krahn, Harvey J., and Graham S. Lowe. 1988. *Work, Industry and Canadian Society.* Scarborough, ON: Nelson Canada.

Lawrence, Bonita. 2004. *"Real Indians" and Others: Mixed Blood Urban Native Peoples and Indigenous Nationhood.* Vancouver: UBC Press.

Lee-Cunin, Marina. 1989. *Daughters of Seacole: A Study of Black Nurses in West Yorkshire.*

Yorkshire: West Yorkshire Low Pay Unit.

Lewis, Stephen. 1992. "The Stephen Lewis Report." Toronto, June 9.

Lum, Janet, and A. Paul Williams. 2000. "Professional Fault Lines: Nursing in Ontario after the Regulated Health Professions Act." In Diana L. Gustafson (ed.), *Care and Consequences: The Impact of Healthcare Reform.* Halifax, NS: Fernwood.

MacDonald, Valerie. 1995. Letter to Linda Ackroyd, Ontario Human Rights Commission, Toronto. June 2.

Makropoulos, Josee. 2004. "Speak White!" In Camille A. Nelson, et al. (eds.), *Racism, Eh? A Critical Inter-Disciplinary Anthology of Race and Racism in Canada.* Concord, ON: Captus Press.

Marx, Karl. 1967. *Capital. Vol. 1.* New York: International Publishers.

Maylor, David. 1987. "SA-Born Nurse Fights For Rights." *Share* 9 (42): 1.

McClintock, Anne. 1995. *Imperial Leather: Gender and Sexuality in the Colonial Contest.* New York: Routledge.

McCloskey, Joanne Comi, and Helen Kennedy Grace. 1997. "Diversity in Nursing: A Formidable Challenge." In Joanne Comi McCloskey and Helen Kennedy Grace (eds.), *Current Issues in Nursing.* St. Louis: Mosby Year Book.

McIntosh, Peggy. 1990. "White Privilege: Unpacking the Invisible Knapsack." *Independent Schools* Winter.

McKenzie, Kwame. 2003. "Editorials: Racism and Health." Available at <http://bmj.com:80/cgi/content/full/326/7380/65> accessed February 16, 2003.

Mensah, Joseph. 2002. *Black Canadians: History, Experiences, Social Conditions.* Halifax, NS: Fernwood Publishing.

Miles, Robert. 1989. *Racism.* London and New York: Routledge.

Miles, Robert, and Rudy Torres. 1996. "Does 'Race' Matter? Transatlantic Perspectives on Racism after 'Race Relations.'" In Vered Amit-Talai and Caroline Knowles (eds.), *Re-Situating Identities: The Politics of Race, Ethnicity, Culture.* Canada: Broadview Press.

Minority Nurse Editors. 2001. "Minority Nurse Population: Going Up!" *Vital Signs* July.

Montagu, Ashley. 1951. *Statement on Race.* New York: Henry Schuman

Murray, Maureen. 1991. Blacks Call for Action after Riot in Halifax. *Toronto Star* July: A1.

Murray, Michael, and Angela Frisina. 1988. *Nursing Morale in Toronto: An Analysis of Career, Job, and Hospital Satisfaction Among Hospital Staff Nurses.* Prepared for the Nursing Manpower Task Force of the Hospital Council of Metropolitan Toronto. September.

Murray, Michael, and Susan Smith. 1988. *Nurses Resigning Their Hospital Jobs in Toronto: Who Are They, Why Are They Resigning, and What Are They Going to Do?* Prepared for the Nursing Manpower Task Force of the Hospital Council of Metropolitan Toronto. August.

Muszynski, Leon, and Jeffrey Reitz. 1982. "Racial and Ethnic Discrimination in Employment." Working Paper #5. Social Planning Council of Metro Toronto. February.

Nestel, Sheryl. 2000. *Obstructed Labour: Race and Gender in the Re-Emergence of Midwifery in Ontario.* Phd thesis, University of Toronto.

Ng, Roxana. 2002. "Freedom from Whom? Globalization and Trade from the

Standpoint of Garment Workers." *Canadian Woman Studies* 21/22 (4 & 1) 74–81.

Nova Scotia Advisory Group on Race Relations. 1991. *Report of the Nova Scotia Advisory Group on Race Relations.* Halifax, Nova Scotia.

Nova Scotia Court of Appeal. 1995. *Regina v. R.D.S.*, October 25.

Ogilvie, Megan. 2008 "Nursing Crisis Worse Than Ever." *Toronto Star* June 14: A19.

Omi, Michael, and Howard Winant. 1994. *Racial Formation in the United States.* New York and London: Routledge.

Ontario Federation of Labour. 1981. "Statement on Racism Hurts Everyone." *Racism Hurts Everyone Kit.* Nov. 23–26.

Ontario Human Rights Commission (OHRC). 2005. "Policy and Guidelines on Racism and Racial Discrimination." June 9.

_____. 2001. *Policy on Racial Slurs and Harassment and Racial Jokes.* Queen's Printer for Ontario.

_____. 1997. Letter to College of Nurses of Ontario ("CNO") Decision Regarding Graduate Nurses. October 23. Toronto.

ONA (Ontario Nurses Association). 1997. "Proxy Pay Equity: Backgrounder." Available at <http://www.ona.org/Political_Act/Curr_Issues/backgrounder.htm> accessed Jan. 1, 1997.

_____. 1999. "Downtown Toronto Health Workers Censure University Health Network." Available at <http://www.newswire.ca/releases/December1999/o8/c2235.html> accessed April 2, 2002.

ONA Vision. 2005. 32, 2 (Spring).

_____. 2002. 29, 1 (Winter).

Ontario Women's Directorate. 1994. *Workplace Harassment: An Action Guide For Women.* Toronto: Ontario Women's Directorate.

Ornstein, Michael. 2006. *Ethno-Racial Groups in Toronto, 1971–2001: A Demographic and Socio-Economic Profile.* Institute for Social Research, York University. January.

Pottins, Melanie. 2000. "Equity Issues: Reaching Out to Aboriginal Members." *ONA Vision* Spring.

Romanow, Roy. 2003. "Executive Summary." Commission on the Future of Health Care in Canada. Ottawa.

Rosen, Rachel. 2001. "Filipino Nurses in Canada." *Canadian Women's Health Network Magazine* 4 (3) Spring. Available at <http://www.cwhn.ca/network-reseau/4-3pg7.html> accessed April 2, 2002.

Rosenberg, Janet, Harry Perlstadt and Willima R.F. Phillips. 2002. "'Now That We Are Here': Discrimination, Disparagement, and Harassment at Work and the Experience of Women Lawyers." In Paula Dubeck amd Dana Dunn (eds.), *Workplace/Women's Place: An Anthology.* Los Angeles: Roxbury Publishing Company.

Samuelson, Wayne. 2002. "OFL Backs Need for More Nurses." *ONA Vision* 29 (1).

Small, Peter. 2004. "Judge Raps Police in 'Driving While Black' Case." *Toronto Star* Friday, September 17: A1.

Smith, Dorothy E. 1992. "Feminist Reflections on Political Economy." In M. Patricia Connelly and Pat Armstrong (eds.), *Feminism in Action: Studies in Political Economy.* Toronto: Canadian Scholars' Press.

Solomos, John, and Les Back. 1996. *Racism and Society.* New York: St. Martin's Press.

Spears, John. 1991. "Africville Won't Die, Blacks Vow." *Toronto Star* July 29: A14.

Stasiulis, Daiva. 1999. "Feminist Intersectional Theorizing." In Peter S. Li (ed.), *Race and Ethnic Relations in Canada*. Toronto: Oxford University Press.

Statistics Canada. 2000. "Women in Canada 2000: A Gender-Based Statistical Report." p.10–14. Ottawa.

_____. 2003. "Ethnic Diversity Survey: Portrait of a Multicultural Society." September. Ottawa: Minister of Industry.

Stevenson, Winona. 1999. "Colonialism and First Nations Women in Canada." In Enakshi Dia and Angela Robertson (eds.), *Scratching the Surface: Canadian Anti-Racist Feminist Thought*." Toronto: Women's Press.

Taylor, Lesley Ciarula. 2008. "Steady Work Drew Nurses to U.S., Study Finds." *Toronto Star* Sept. 30: A15.

Teelucksingh, Cheryl, and Grace-Edward Galabuzi. 2005. "Working Precariously: The Impact of Race and Immigrant Status on Employment Opportunities and Outcomes in Canada." *Directions* 2, 1: 15–52.

Thornhill, Esmeralda. 1991. "Focus on Black Women." In Jesse Vorst et al. (eds.), *Race, Class, Gender: Bonds and Barriers*. Winnipeg: Society for Socialist Studies.

Toronto Star. 2002a. "An Investigation into Race and Crime." October 19: A1.

_____. 2002b. "Race and Crime." October 20: A1.

_____ 2003. "Worth Repeating: Good Healthcare Needs Full-Time Nurses." May 13: A22.

_____. 2005. "Editorial: Revolving Door at Hospitals." Jan. 23: A16.

Urquhart, Ian. 2003. "Facing Up to Reality on Nurses." *Toronto Star* May 12: A19.

Van Dijk, Teun. 1993. *Elite Discourse and Racism*. Newbury Park: Sage Publications

Vosko, Leah F. 2000. *Temporary Work: The Gendered Rise of a Precarious Employment Relationship*. Toronto: University of Toronto.

Wahl, Barb. 2002. Letter to Mr. Keith C. Norton, Ontario Human Rights Commission. Jan. 4.

Walker, James W. St. G. 1985. *Racial Discrimination in Canada: The Black Experience*. Ottawa: Canadian Historical Association.

Welsh, Sandy, et al. 2001. "When You Depend on Your Workplace for Your Livelihood, You Can't Walk Away: The Experience of Women who Reported Sexual Harassment." In Geri Sanson and Mark Hart (eds.), *Responding to Harassment and Discrimination: Key Issues and Effective Strategies*. Professional Development Program, Osgoode Hall Law School of York University.

Winkelmann-Gleed, Andrea. 2007. "Gender, International Recruitment and Migration of Public Service Workers with Implications for the Management of Equality and Diversity." Paper for the 5th International Disciplinary Conference, London, UK, June.

Wortley, Scott, and Julian Tanner. 2003. "Data, Denials and Confusion: The Racial Profile Debate in Toronto." *Canadian Journal of Criminology and Criminal Justice* 45: 367–89.

Zeltric, Claire. 2002. "Nursing Shortage Is About a Lot More than Numbers." *Toronto Star* Aug. 21: A19.